D0592793

Dr. Rechtschaffen's Diet
for Lifetime Weight Control
and Better Health

Dr. Rechtschaffen's

Diet

for Lifetime Weight Control and Better Health

Joseph S. Rechtschaffen, M.D.
and Robert Carola

With original recipes by Ann Seranne

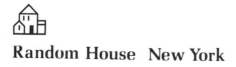

Random House New York

Copyright © 1980 by Joseph S. Rechtschaffen, M.D.,
and Robert Carola
All rights reserved under International and Pan-American
Copyright Conventions.
Published in the United States by Random House, Inc.,
New York and simultaneously in Canada by Random
House of Canada Limited, Toronto.

Library of Congress Cataloging in Publication Data
Rechtschaffen, Joseph S
Dr. Rechtschaffen's Diet for Lifetime Weight Control
and Better Health
Includes index.
1. Reducing diets—Recipes. 2. Reducing diets.
I. Carola, Robert, joint author. II. Seranne, Ann.
III. Title. IV. Title: Diet for lifetime weight
control and better health.
RM222.2.R42 1980   613.2'5   80–5302
ISBN 0–394–51188–3

Manufactured in the United States of America
9 8 7 6 5 4 3 2
First Edition

To our wives,
Fran and Leslie

Contents

Acknowledgments

The authors would like to thank Craig Claiborne
for his help and for demonstrating so vividly by
his own example that the Rechtschaffen Diet
works. He has been a good friend and a model
patient. We would also like to thank Michael
Tong, co-owner of Shun Lee Palace Restaurant,
and Adi Giovannetti and John Lonzar, co-owners
of Il Nido, Il Monello, Il Minestrello, and Piccolo
Mondo for their generous cooperation. Finally,
we are indebted to Charlotte Mayerson, our
editor at Random House, for her unerring taste
and skill.

Dr. Rechtschaffen's Diet
for Lifetime Weight Control
and Better Health

Introduction

The Power of
Positive Eating

I have been a doctor since 1945, and I've seen a lot of people try a lot of different diets since then. Good nutrition has always been one of my main interests, and somewhere along the way I realized that it made much more sense to prevent disease than just to treat it. There was no conscious decision, and no specific time when I stopped doing one thing and started doing another.

I knew that if I was really interested in treating the *whole* person, I had to do more than just be a doctor of internal medicine and a specialist in gastroenterology (the study of the digestive system). I knew that if I wanted to treat people so that they would understand that good health is normal, I had to involve them in a new lifestyle. Of course, that included what they eat.

And as I became more and more involved with diet and nutrition, I became more and more aware of a disease that most

of us took for granted—a disease that was spreading throughout the country and even the world, a disease that struck
young, old, rich and poor. That disease is obesity—being overweight.

I have read statistics that say that 30 million Americans are
overweight. Other statistics claim that as many as 70 million
Americans are overweight. Let's compromise and say that
there are 50 million Americans who weigh more than they
should. More than they would like to.

Using past history as a guide, it's safe to say that most
overweight people are on a diet, have been on a diet, or will
go on a diet. People don't usually go on one diet and stop there.
They keep trying—10, 12, 15, 20 different diets. Once in a
while a diet works *permanently*, and the quest for a new lifestyle ends happily. But more than likely, if you've tried twenty
diets you'll try the twenty-first one also.

Obviously, something is wrong.

You are in control of your life—no one else. You can make
good things happen if you want them to. How? By being
positive. By *knowing* that you really are in control. By not
giving up—even when you might have a reason to be discouraged.

Positive thinking is important, but so is positive eating.
You don't get thin and *stay* thin by starving yourself. You get
thin and *stay* thin by eating properly. By eating positively.

For a long time now you've been thinking about what *not*
to eat. Now you can start thinking about what *to* eat.

I love to eat as much as you do, and I'm not about to
prescribe a diet for you that I wouldn't follow myself. The
Rechtschaffen Diet is a program that actually encourages eating. It asks you to think about what you eat and *how* you eat
it. It gives you a chance to live a normal life with the emphasis
on acceptance, not rejection.

The Rechtschaffen Diet asks you to cut down on salt, simple sugars and fats. At the same time, it recommends that you eat *more* complex-sugars (carbohydrates) such as vegetables and whole-grain, and *more* high-fiber foods such as leafy vegetables, unpeeled raw fruits and unprocessed miller's bran. (From here on we'll use the term "residue" instead of "fiber.")

It is possible that you will eat more on my diet than you are eating now. The big difference is that you will try not to eat the foods that will add pounds and also be harmful to your body in other ways.

No one on my diet feels deprived. You won't miss what you give up, and you won't give up anything permanently. You will eat three meals a day—three *real* meals—and you will be introduced to a realistic and healthy weight-loss plan that will make you feel better, look better, and think better.

You do not have to stop eating any foods permanently. You do not have to disrupt your life.

You will lose weight and keep it off if you can think of your diet as something that you honestly want to do. That's why the Rechtschaffen Diet works—it is a diet for people who love food and want to keep enjoying it.

If you can make up your mind that being thin and healthy and *having* food is better than being fat and *craving* food, then you can make a positive move to change your lifestyle and lose weight permanently.

If you want to stop being a statistic, there's no one stopping you. If you want to be thin and still eat three rewarding meals a day, no one is stopping you. If you want to lead a full and happy life, go ahead. Times have changed. No one is stopping you.

Chapter 1

What Makes You Fat?

Why Are Some People
Fatter Than Others?

One of the most common cries of the frustrated dieter sounds something like this: "He eats so much and never gains an ounce—I just *look* at a piece of cake and I gain five pounds!" It would be easy to tell such a person that it isn't true. "It's all in your mind." "Go home and think thin." "Stop cheating and start counting calories."

But it *is* true. Some people gain weight very easily and have an almost impossible time losing weight. And there is a clear difference between how men and women gain or lose weight. But just because some people gain weight easily and have trouble losing it doesn't mean they have to *remain* overweight. It doesn't mean they have to be hungry all the time either.

Is Fatness Inherited?

I have heard many of my patients repeat this lament: "Both parents are fat, and all of my brothers and sisters are fat—even my cousins are fat. I guess I'm just meant to be fat too!" Actually, we're still not sure how much truth there is to that sad assessment. What *does* seem certain is that a fat child will grow up to be a fat adult.

On the surface it appears that fatness is inherited, because fat parents usually have fat children (when both parents are obese, 75 percent of the children will also be obese), but there may be other reasons for family fatness. Very often, fat parents will feed their children too much food from the time the children are born. If children are taught to overeat while they are very young, the chances are that there will be no turning away from future obesity. It is now thought that a child's fat cells develop during its crucial first two years. Once fat cells become overabundant by a pattern of overeating, the number of cells always remains higher than normal.

I once met a young overweight mother who asked my advice about her new baby. When I suggested that she talk with her pediatrician, she told me she already had, but was merely curious about my opinion. It seems that the baby was vomiting frequently and would not eat as much as the mother thought he should. (The fact that the baby continued to gain weight did not seem to impress the mother.) At each meal she kept feeding the child even after the baby signaled that he had had enough, and invariably the baby vomited while he was being fed.

Under the circumstances it was not difficult to predict the mother's answer when I asked her what she did after the baby vomited. "Well," she said, "when he loses all of his food I just start feeding him all over again." I suggested as patiently as I could that perhaps she was forcing the baby to eat more than he really needed. Her eyes opened wide in surprise but she did not cut back on the baby's intake of food. Is it any wonder that the little boy grew up to be an overweight adolescent with all the extra problems that fat teenagers have?

Although obesity itself may not be a totally inherited factor, it is likely that the *potential* to be fat *is* inherited. However, a child who has the potential to be fat doesn't necessarily have to *be* fat. If a child is active and doesn't overeat, the chances are good that he or she will remain lean. In contrast, a child raised in a family situation where too much food is eaten and physical activity is minimized will probably become overweight.

Is Your "Stop" Signal Working?

People who are obese, or who have the genetic potential to be obese, seem to overeat when they are emotionally upset. Not only will obese people overeat when they are stimulated, but they will have trouble stopping. The cause of such compulsive eating under stress is not fully understood but it has been studied enough to be taken seriously as a real phenomenon.

One of my patients knows she is overweight and says she would like to stop being overweight, but she keeps on eating long after most people would be satisfied.

Though we don't really think about it or notice it, most of us get a signal when we have eaten enough to satisfy our hunger. This is sometimes called a "satisfaction response." Some overweight people have lost the ability to respond to their satisfaction response. They don't notice the signal to stop eating anymore. As strange as it may sound to you if you don't have a similar problem, a faulty appetite-control center is an awful reality for many people who tend to become overweight.

What can you do if your satisfaction response doesn't work anymore? It usually takes a strong will and the determination to create a new lifestyle to overcome a faulty satisfaction response. You simply must condition yourself to think about the *amount* of food you are eating. You may still feel hungry after eating a full meal of recommended portions of good food, but if you try to be honest about it, you will admit that you don't need any more food for a while.

If you don't put too much food on your plate to begin with (and don't go back for seconds), you stand a pretty good chance of reactivating a dormant satisfaction response.

Can You Blame Your Hormones?

In case you are wondering how often obesity is caused by hormonal or other medical problems, it appears that such cases occur less than 5 percent of the time.

Although most fat people may not have hormonal problems, they do have some body differences that keep them overweight. For instance, fat people usually have high amounts of insulin in their blood—most often caused by what they eat. The insulin encourages obesity by helping to convert sugar into fat quickly, and by helping the sugar get into the fat cell in the first place. On top of this, the increased insulin secreted by fat people may actually be an appetite stimulant. So not only do fat people have more than the usual desire to eat, but the food that is eaten is rapidly converted into fat.

One of the ways to cope with this problem is to eat slowly. The faster you eat, the faster your insulin will act on sugar and use it to manufacture fat. Also, two or three small meals will cause less insulin to be secreted than one very large meal, so avoid the once-a-day dinner gorging that is supposed to make up for the skipped breakfast and lunch. It doesn't work that way. Eat all three meals, but keep the portions small.

Remember, just because you have a tendency to gain weight doesn't mean you *have* to gain weight. Don't blame your genes, your insulin or your fat cells. There are two main causes of fatness: overeating and lack of exercise.

And also remember this: Just because *you* are fat (at least temporarily) *doesn't mean your children have to be fat.* Keep your children thin, and spare them the pain and embarrassment you have felt.

Dieting Differences
Between Men and Women

Not only do some individuals have more weight problems than other people, most women gain weight more easily than men. And once a woman gains weight she has more trouble losing it than a man does. A recent study in East Germany showed that twice as many women as men were overweight. Why are more women than men overweight? Why do women have so much trouble losing weight? Can women follow the same diet that men can? Women are definitely *not* the same as men. The differences range from hormonal to physical to social.

Physical Differences   One reason why men lose weight about twice as fast as women is that they have extra muscle tissue which burns off twice as many calories as fat does—and women's bodies have a high proportion of fat to muscle. There is very little a woman can do to alter her basic muscle-to-fat proportions, except not to add *more* fat.

Actually, a woman's fatty padding acts as an emergency food reservoir which can provide food for the fetus if, for some reason, the pregnant mother-to-be is without food for a short time.

Unfortunately, just because women are usually smaller and less muscular than men doesn't mean they have smaller appetites. There is usually very little difference between the appetites of men and women.

Hormonal Differences   A friend of mine who teaches biology at Barnard College in New York City once said this about the anatomy of women: "Compared with the intricate workings of the female sexual system, a moon rocket is a simple toy." And that complexity of a woman's body explains a great deal about women's dieting differences and problems.

Most of my patients lose about 2 pounds a week after the first week or so on the diet. That is a good, rapid rate. But for a woman, a steady weight loss of 2 pounds a week is almost always upset one week out of every month. The week in question is the one just before the start of the menstrual period. During that week there is virtually nothing a woman can do to keep her weight down, and most women are lucky if they don't actually *gain* weight during that week.

Weight gain just before the onset of the menstrual period is caused by the retention of fluids in the body. Salt enhances fluid retention, and the more salt you use the more fluid weight you will gain.

Female hormones are essential for the maintenance of

female traits and for the proper working of the entire female sexual cycle that makes it possible for women to have babies. Unfortunately for the female dieter, female hormones also produce and store fat. There is no denying that the female hormones—estrogen and progesterone—make it more difficult for a woman to stay thin. Even synthetic female hormones such as those used in birth-control pills will cause weight gain.

There is no ready solution to a woman's hormonal complications. The best she can do is understand that along with the premenstrual tension and irritability, there may be at that time of the month a craving for sweets, bloating of the intestinal tract and breasts, and insatiable hunger. Obviously, for those days, there will be no way your diet will work properly. Make it easier for yourself by avoiding salt and the worst of the fattening foods; know that as soon as your period starts you will be able to resume an effective program of weight loss—at least for the next three weeks until the monthly cycle starts all over again.

Chapter 2

What Do Diets Do?

Most people who have been on a diet will tell you that it's not really difficult to lose weight—at least temporarily. "It's easy," they say. "I've done it lots of times." It's true, isn't it? You can stop smoking, or lose weight, or just about anything, for a week or two—but can you lose weight, and keep it off, once and for all?

Why Do People Go on Diets?

Most diets have the same goal: weight loss. Many diet programs become popular because they promise a *quick* weight loss—just in time for your class reunion, or your sister's wedding, or your summer vacation in a trim new bathing suit. But a very rapid weight loss can be an unhealthy jolt for your body. It is always preferable to take weight off slowly and *keep it off.* (Best of all, don't gain weight in the first place.) If you have lost weight and gained it back, and repeated that process over and over again, you have probably done more harm to your body than if you had remained overweight to begin with.

Every year, Americans spend billions of dollars in an effort to lose weight. About $90 million is spent on diet aids that do not need prescriptions, and another $54 million is spent on drugs that are prescribed by physicians. If you can afford it, you may visit an exclusive health spa, where another $220 million is spent every year by hopeful dieters.

These figures are not surprising when we realize that about 50 million Americans (most of them women over forty years old) are overweight. The average American adult has tried 10 or 15 diets, usually staying on none of them more than three months. Most dieters expect miracles but find only that losing weight is simply a matter of eating less fattening food and exercising more. That doesn't sound like much fun, so they wait until the next miracle diet or miracle drug comes along.

"Miracle diets" may be harmful—many do not provide well-balanced meals—and "miracle drugs" are potentially just as dangerous.

What Do Diet Pills Do?

Apparently, diet pills and other diet drugs *can* help you lose weight, at least during a short initial burst, but the side effects are not worth it, especially because the lost weight may not really be permanently lost at all.

Prescription diet pills are usually amphetamines, or amphetamine-related. Small doses of amphetamines do not remain effective for long, and their continued use may cause addiction or mental stress. Many other diet pills can be obtained without prescription. These usually contain benzocaine and phenylpropanolamine (PPA). Benzocaine is a well-known painkiller (sometimes found in cough drops or anti-itch insect sprays) that is supposed to dull the taste buds, and PPA has been used often in nose drops as a nasal decongestant.

The problem with drugs such as PPA is their potential side effects. PPA may aggravate cases of high blood pressure and other heart-related diseases, diabetes, and thyroid disease, exactly those maladies that often plague overweight people in the first place. When dieters swallow nonprescription diet drugs they risk the possibility of side effects that could be fatal.

Another form of drug therapy uses diuretics, drugs that stimulate urination in order to eliminate salt and water. Diuretics do nothing toward eliminating fat, however, and any weight loss is strictly temporary. As usual with diet drugs, side effects are prominent, including nausea and dizziness because of the excessive loss of sodium and potassium.

Other drugs such as thyroid hormone do not produce a permanent loss of weight either, and can be harmful to people with any form of heart disease, including high blood pressure. Such hormone remedies, when they are not specifically prescribed for hormonal problems, usually upset the body's delicate balance. Such imbalances are frequently more difficult to treat than obesity.

An interesting sidelight on diet pills is that patients who are given placebos (harmless, inactive pills) usually lose just as much weight as they do with real diet pills. The basic principle of placebos underlies the entire field of dieting: If a person is motivated to lose weight, almost any change in eating style will accomplish a short-term result that makes the dieter happy. Diets that allow you to eat only small quantities of one type of food (carbohydrates, proteins or fats) will probably change your ordinary routine sufficiently so that you actually will lose weight for a short time.

●

What Are Some of the Other Problems with Diets?

The most obvious fault of most diets is their inability to help you lose weight permanently. Fad diets may *get* you thin, but they won't *keep* you thin.

It stands to reason that a firmly regimented diet that consistently deprives you of food is not going to work for long. If a diet program is too rigid, telling you exactly what and when to eat, it is almost impossible to leave your house without being inconvenienced or going off the diet altogether. You certainly won't look forward to going to restaurants, where everyone else seems to be (and probably is) eating better than you are.

The average person on a diet loses weight almost immediately, but quickly becomes bored with the monotony of the diet and soon decides that being fat is better than being bored. After a month or two, the old habits return and the diet is over. After all, you say, you don't want to be constantly reminded that you have to be on a diet.

One of the most harmful things that any diet can do is to take away foods that you need to be healthy. Your diet must provide a well-balanced, nutritious program, otherwise you are flirting with sickness or even death. Many people on high-something, low-everything-else diets have complained of being sluggish, irritable and sexually impotent. Their skin and hair become dry and brittle, they become constipated because high-residue foods are decreased, and they smoke more because they have to put *something* into their mouths! Blood cholesterol can go up, and malnutrition may become a reality.

Hunger from dieting is extremely dangerous. A hungry person—one who is used to eating large quantities of food and who is consciously being deprived of food—can easily go on a wild eating binge. The binge leads to a weight gain, which leads to feelings of frustration, depression and failure, which lead to another binge. If your diet is going to be successful, you should not be hungry all the time. Nobody can be expected to cope with constant hunger.

Potential Problems
with Specific Types of Diets

Low-carbohydrate diets deprive you of vital carbohydrates, causing headaches, tiredness and dizziness. Such a diet places an extra burden on the kidneys and may produce kidney failure, which can be fatal; it may also produce gout because of the increased urea in the blood. Typically, low-carbohydrate diets stimulate a quick weight loss, but just as typically, the loss is water, not body fat.

A pregnant woman should never go on any kind of diet without the approval and supervision of her physician. One of the possible side effects for a pregnant woman on a low-carbohydrate diet is brain damage to the unborn baby. Actually, anyone with a health problem should check with a physician before starting a diet.

Liquid protein diets can be very dangerous. As many as fifty deaths may have been caused by liquid protein diets. Such a diet does not provide the essential amino acids the body needs to build its protein—the deprivation strains the body and causes a severe imbalance in the overall diet. The liquid protein diets are so unbalanced that the list of possible problems is long: kidney stones, gout, hair loss, tiredness, dizziness, nausea, headaches, bad breath, poor circulation and difficulty keeping warm, dry skin, constipation, menstrual irregularity, gall-bladder disturbances, irregular heartbeat and even cardiac arrest. Many of the more serious problems seem to occur when dieters stop the diet. Apparently, the change in the body's metabolism causes an exaggerated strain on the heart that can be disastrous.

Fasting and *advanced macrobiotic* diets can literally starve you to death. An advanced macrobiotic diet, which recommends only rice, for example, or complete fasting, robs you of essential nutrients and can cause severe malnutrition, protein deficiency, and kidney, intestinal, and heart disorders. Prolonged fasting or the exclusive intake of only one food that merely fills your stomach may ultimately lead to mental disorders and death.

What Does a "Good" Diet Do?

A "good" diet program reduces calories moderately but still provides a well-balanced menu. It employs exercise and changes your lifestyle so that the diet works permanently. It doesn't promise short-term miracles, and doesn't produce any. A proper diet will show you how to keep the extra weight off without depriving you of the basic pleasure of eating and enjoying good food.

A sensible diet produces a steady weight loss of about two pounds a week instead of a more dramatic initial weight loss that is probably only water anyway.

If a diet is going to work, you have to be able to live with it. You should never have to feel uncomfortable or unprepared when you dine in a restaurant or at someone else's home. A "good" diet is flexible enough to fit into the real world.

"Junk" Foods, "Fast" Foods
and "Health" Foods

The U.S. Department of Agriculture recently defined "junk food" as a food of "minimal nutritional value." It's even worse than that. Not only do foods such as soft drinks, candy, potato chips and chewing gum provide almost no basic nutrients, they are also downright harmful to your body. Nevertheless, America's favorite "food" is the canned soft drink. The average American drinks about 400 cans of soft drinks in a year! That's 225 percent more than in 1950. (Try making your own "soda pop" by adding fresh or unsweetened fruit juice to low-salt mineral water or club soda. It actually tastes better than commercial soft drinks, and it will quench your thirst faster.)

Americans spend over $100 billion a year on processed foods, including ready-to-eat convenience foods and snacks of all kinds. We spend almost *half* of our food money on high-convenience, low-nutrition foods. And the processed food industry is growing rapidly, very rapidly.

Food companies have solved the problems of packaging and preserving food that stays fresh for weeks or even months on a supermarket shelf. The food business has become the chemistry business. Today it is the scientists, not the cooks, who are appealing to our tastes. They can make it saltier, sweeter, pinker or whatever it is that is "in" that week.

Our favorite meat is beef. Almost half of the beef we consume goes into fast-food hamburgers. Our favorite vegetable is the frozen French fry. That's an astonishing list of favorite foods! We are eating the all-American meal: hamburger, French fries and soda. We couldn't be eating much worse.

One of the reasons why Americans eat and drink so many

fattening "empty calories" is that "junk food" tastes the way they are conditioned to want it to. It's usually loaded with either salt or sugar—two of the most harmful foods in our diets. Another reason is that television commercials for low-nutrition foods are extremely effective. The average child sees over 10,000 food commercials every year and about $600 million is spent annually on television advertising for children. According to a Harvard Business School study, a mother buys the cereal her child wants about 88 percent of the time. Obviously the commercials are successful.

Eating patterns are set early. Some well-meaning parents make "food junkies" of their children by rewarding them with salt and sugar in one gaudy package or another. Don't call junk foods "treats." A treat should be something that is good for you. Snacks filled with large amounts of sugar and salt may very well be setting the stage in American schoolchildren for later problems with high blood pressure and atherosclerosis.

In 1970 school lunches for our children contained more saturated fats than the average American diet did, and it was not until 1976 that at least one baby-food manufacturer stopped putting sugar in fruit juices. In 1977, under pressure from consumers and authorities alike, salt was no longer added to baby foods. In both cases, sales did not decrease.

No one is born with a preference for salt—it is an acquired taste. The salt was being added to suit the mother's palate, not the baby's.

In addition to the packaged convenience foods they consume, more Americans are eating at inexpensive fast-food restaurants than ever before, and they are eating high-fat, high-sugar, low-nutrition food. Americans spend about $20 billion a year at fast-food chains. One of the leading fast-food chains sells about two *billion* hamburgers a year, and it is estimated that in five years Americans will eat half of their meals away from home—presumably in the same kind of places, eating the same kind of "empty calorie" food.

As for "health foods," that trend may indeed be healthy. There seems to be a genuine concern growing for good nutrition (a recent poll showed that almost 90 percent of adult Americans wanted to find out more about nutrition), and many excellent foods are now available that eliminate sugar, salt and other questionable ingredients. It should be noted, however, that some "health foods" merely substitute one problem food for another, or merely charge extra for placing the word "natural" on the label. For example, "sea salt" may sound pure and fresh and natural, but it's still sodium chloride—the same as table salt. Honey may sound more "natural" than sugar—but its food value is basically the same.

Learn to read labels, and make sure you really know what you are eating and drinking. Nowadays it seems as if you need an advanced degree in chemistry to be able to make sense out of most labels, but even if most of the chemical ingredients read like gobbledygook (they are usually preservatives or artificial coloring and flavoring—sometimes referred to as "flavor enhancers"), there are a few things you can learn.

First of all, you can tell whether the food contains such simple ingredients as salt, sugar, butter or white flour. You can also find out what *type* of oil or other shortenings have been used. By checking the order in which ingredients are listed you can also get a general idea of the amount of any ingredient. For instance, if sugar is listed first and salt is listed second, the food contains more sugar than salt. Unfortunately, you can't tell how *much* of any ingredient is used.

Chapter 3

What Are the Benefits of the Rechtschaffen Diet?

What Is the Rechtschaffen Diet?

The Rechtschaffen Diet is a low-salt,* low-simple-sugar, low-fat, high-carbohydrate, high-residue† diet. Notice that I said *low-*salt, *low-*sugar, *low-*fat—not *no-*salt, *no-*sugar, *no-*fat. I cannot stress this point enough. After you have been on the Rechtschaffen Diet for four weeks and have achieved a distinc-

---

*What's wrong with salt? Salt has been definitely connected to high blood pressure and other cardiovascular diseases. The intake of excessive salt also increases fluid retention, premenstrual tension and abdominal bloating. Salt causes you to gain weight. The average adult needs 2–3 grams of salt per day—this amount is satisfied in the Rechtschaffen Diet. In contrast, the average American adult consumes about 30 grams of salt each day—about 10 times more than the body needs. If you are taking lithium, you need some sodium to avoid any toxic effects. If you are taking lithium, consult your physician to determine how much salt you need in your daily diet.

†*What is residue?* Residue is also known as fiber, bulk or roughage. We use the term "residue" because it best describes the true nature of the food. Residue means "what is left over," and the residue in foods consists of material that the body cannot digest—the residue is left over after digestion is complete. Residue is found only in plants, not in meat, poultry or fish. Unprocessed miller's bran is the most practical form of residue, and other good sources are whole grains, leafy vegetables and raw fruits with skin. Foods do not necessarily have to be stringy and crunchy to contain residue.

tive weight loss that satisfies you, you are free to eat additional foods in moderation.

In February 1980 the United States government issued the first federal dietary guidelines ever. The guidelines were published jointly by the Department of Agriculture and the Department of Health, Education and Welfare. The guidelines, which may be the first step toward a national policy on nutrition, *coincide with principles of the Rechtschaffen Diet in every way*.

The guidelines specify:

1. Eat a variety of foods.
2. Maintain ideal weight.
3. Avoid too much fat, saturated fat and cholesterol.
4. Eat foods with adequate starch [complex-sugar carbohydrates] and fiber [residue].
5. Avoid too much sugar.
6. Avoid too much sodium [salt].
7. If you drink alcohol, do so in moderation.

One of the most dramatic features of the Rechtschaffen Diet is the emphasis on a high-carbohydrate, high-residue diet. Just about every other diet recommends low salt, low simple sugar and low fat. Very few diets recommend high *anything*, with the possible exception of protein.

It is very important to cut down on calories and other unwanted ingredients by severely reducing your intake of salt, simple sugars and fats. Just about any doctor will tell you that. What they may not tell you is that it is just as important to eat a *high*-carbohydrate, *high*-residue diet to lose weight, feel better and be healthier. The *combination* of high carbohydrates and high residue is especially important. Both features are good by themselves, but together they become more than twice as effective.

The difference in the Rechtschaffen Diet is not only what you *don't* eat, but also what you *do* eat. It is an active diet of *eating,* not of starving or of deprivation. It is a diet that helps you live the way you were supposed to.

After all, human beings did not always eat everything. Originally we ate grains and other vegetables that gave us a high-carbohydrate, high-residue diet. We did not learn to eat a "modern" diet that includes large amounts of salt, sugar and fat until recently—and it has been only recently in our history that our problems with our diets have begun.

I have found that people on the Rechtschaffen Diet usually lose about 2 pounds a week after the first week. You can actually lose up to 10 pounds the first week because so much of it is merely extra fluid. But think of the typical pace as 2 pounds a week. Some diets promise 10 or even 20 pounds a week—and they may even deliver, at least for a couple of weeks or so. But what happens after that? Slowly but surely, the weight returns.

One of my patients proved to be a model of consistency. When she first consulted me she weighed 179 pounds. After a series of tests she started on my diet and exercise program, and after the first month she had lost 10 pounds. After three months she had lost 21 pounds, after six months she had lost 36½ pounds, and after a full year she had lost exactly 40 pounds—and she continued to lose. In no week did she lose more than 4 pounds, but she never became discouraged, and except for a clambake and one or two holiday dinners, she never seriously went off the diet.

Most overweight people are in a hurry. It may have taken five years or more to gain their extra weight, but they want to lose it in time for cousin Linda's wedding two weeks from now.

I want you to lose weight *permanently.* You want the same thing. Go on a crash diet and lose weight in time for Linda's wedding if you must, but come back to a plan that can keep you slim *and* healthy for the rest of your life.

Be patient. If you lose 2 pounds a week, you will lose 25 pounds in only three months, and *you will keep it off.* You will lose about 2 pounds a week for as long as you need to. Your body has a built-in "normal" weight. You will level off at that weight and then maintain it by adjusting the Rechtschaffen Diet to suit your personal needs. Chapter 7—"After the First Month . . . Staying on the Diet"—shows you how to maintain your desired weight and still eat whatever you want, at least some of the time.

What Are the Benefits
of the Rechtschaffen Diet?

Naturally most people go on diets to lose weight. That is the most immediate goal, and usually it is the most obvious benefit. If you stay on the Rechtschaffen Diet even most of the time, *you will lose weight.* But losing weight is by no means the only benefit you will receive from the Rechtschaffen Diet.

Heart disease and cancer are America's leading killers. Almost one million Americans will die this year from some form of heart disease. Cancer will claim another 400,000 lives, and that figure is on the rise. Although heart-disease deaths are actually decreasing, the American death rate from heart disease is still one of the highest in the world.

It would be absurd to claim that these 1,400,000 Americans could be saved every year if they merely watched their diets, but it would be equally irresponsible not to point out some obvious connections between diet and disease.

In 1980 the National Conference on Diabetes suggested that a high-carbohydrate, high-residue diet might benefit people with diabetes by reducing their requirement for insulin. In the same year, the Gerontological Society agreed with the recommendations that emerged from the National Conference on Diabetes, and said that a high-carbohydrate, high-residue diet "takes the heat off the pancreas" and permits a more efficient use of the available insulin.

The Rechtschaffen Diet concentrates on introducing the following basic factors into your diet: (1) low salt; (2) low simple sugar; (3) low fat; (4) high carbohydrate; and (5) high residue. It also recommends regular physical activity to ensure the maximum benefits of the diet.

Exercise is essential to help "burn off" calories and to decrease your appetite. If you can't exercise any other way, walk at least six miles a day, including the walking you do around your home or office. If you buy a walking pedometer (about $15) you will soon find out that you have been walking several miles a day already. (Chapter 4 talks about the importance of exercise.)

Let's see how each of these recommendations benefits you.

Low-salt diet

1. Reduces risk of hypertension (high blood pressure).
2. Reduces edema (fluid retention in body tissues).
3. Reduces premenstrual bloating and tension.
4. Permits the natural flavors of food to emerge.
5. Promotes weight loss.

Low-simple-sugar diet

1. Reduces free fatty acids in the blood.
2. Reduces the risk of hypoglycemia.

3. Raises the level of insulin slowly and therefore does not increase levels of blood fats or stimulate the appetite.
4. Reduces the risk of heart disease.
5. Promotes weight loss.

Low-fat diet

1. Reduces risk of cancer.
2. Reduces risk of atherosclerosis (fatty deposits on the inner walls of arteries), the forerunner of heart attacks and strokes.
3. Decreases fluid retention in the body.
4. Enables you to eat more.
5. Promotes weight loss.

High-carbohydrate diet

1. Reduces risk of heart disease.
2. Is generally inexpensive.
3. Satisfies your desire for food before you overeat.
4. Eliminates the desire for fats and simple sugars.
5. Promotes weight loss.
6. Helps diabetics to use insulin more efficiently.

High-residue diet

1. Reduces risk of cancer of the large intestine and rectum.
2. Reduces risk of hemorrhoids, diverticulosis, varicose veins, hiatus hernia, phlebitis and gall-bladder disease.
3. Prevents both constipation and diarrhea.
4. Lowers absorption of fats, thereby lowering blood cholesterol.
5. Reduces risk of heart disease.
6. Promotes weight loss.
7. Helps diabetics use insulin more efficiently.

Exercise

1. Reduces risk of heart disease.
2. Helps promote weight loss; decreases appetite.
3. Creates a feeling of well-being.
4. Motivates you to stop smoking.
5. Helps relieve arthritis and diabetes.
6. Promotes longevity.
7. Increases blood transport to the brain.
8. Relieves effects of stress.

How the Rechtschaffen Diet
Helps Lower the Risk of Cancer

Food residue and cancer   When it comes to the effects of diet on disease, there is still controversy. All we can do is to try to make good judgments based on apparently reliable evidence, even though some doubt remains. But there is *no doubt* in my mind that *a high-residue diet lowers the risk of cancer of the large intestine.*

The residue in foods such as bran, whole grains, leafy vegetables, and raw fruit with skin absorbs a great deal of moisture and adds bulk to your food as the food passes through your intestines. As a result, your stool is larger, you have more frequent bowel movements, you speed up the passage of feces through your large intestine, and you lower the risk of many problems that may arise in your digestive tract, including constipation, hemorrhoids, and cancer of the rectum and large intestine.

The faster the feces pass through the intestine, the less opportunity they will have to affect the delicate lining of the large intestine. Ordinarily, low-residue food is eliminated 2 or

3 days after it is eaten. With a high-residue diet, however, the food is digested in 12 to 18 hours and eliminated within 24 hours.

Rural blacks in Africa, who eat a high-residue diet, and usually have daily bowel movements, do not have a high incidence of cancer of the large intestine. However, when these same people move to an urban environment they eat less residue and increase their risk of cancer of the large intestine.

Constipation is virtually nonexistent with a high-residue diet, and because the diet is self-regulatory it also prevents diarrhea. In other words, *the Rechtschaffen Diet does not disrupt your body;* it allows it to function normally, the way it is supposed to.

One of my most dramatic cases involved a forty-four-year-old man who had suffered with diarrhea since he was thirteen. He had not had a normal bowel movement in thirty-one years! When I suggested a high-residue diet he didn't believe I could be serious—it was exactly the opposite of what every other doctor had told him to eat. He followed the diet I prescribed, and has been having normal, healthy, regular bowel movements ever since. And of course he is enjoying his meals much more than before because he is eating real food again.

If you are over fifty years old, your chances of getting hemorrhoids are about 50–50. When you are constipated you inadvertently cause side effects such as hemorrhoids by straining during defecation. You put too much pressure on your rectum and large intestine and cause the small blood vessels to balloon. When you begin to take the daily 3 to 4 tablespoons of unprocessed bran that I recommend, you will probably do away with constipation, diarrhea and hemorrhoids at the same time.

I could tell you about dozens of people who were benefited

by a high-residue diet, but let me tell you about only three of my patients who used to suffer from hemorrhoids, anal itching and diverticulitis.

The first man, Mr. A, had markedly enlarged hemorrhoids, for which I prescribed a short-term medication. I also put him on my high-residue diet and an exercise program. The hemorrhoids shrank after four days, and we stopped the medication. Mr. A continued the diet, and the hemorrhoids were completely gone five days later and have not returned.

The second case was a little more complicated. For fifteen years Mr. B had been bothered by constant anal itching, which had been unresponsive to drug therapy and two operations. He was scheduled for additional surgery when he consulted me. I put Mr. B on my diet and told him how important it was to concentrate on high-residue foods and his daily supplement of unprocessed bran. After three weeks the itching was gone, and after five months we discontinued his office visits altogether. The third operation never took place.

Mr. C, like Mr. B, was referred to me by his physician just prior to a scheduled operation. The problem here was diverticulitis, a condition where outpockets form like little balloons on the walls of the large intestine and then become inflamed or infected. A high-residue diet helped clear up Mr. C's diverticulitis, and he and his surgeon cheerfully canceled the operation—permanently.

When a person is not receiving enough protein we say that he or she has a protein deficiency, but when a person is not getting enough residue we don't think of it as a deficiency. We should. Too many Americans are suffering from a deficiency of residue that can be corrected rather easily. Next to water, unprocessed bran is probably your best diet bargain. One pound of unprocessed bran costs about fifty cents and lasts a month.

Besides helping to avoid many gastrointestinal problems, 3 to 4 tablespoons of bran each day will help you lose weight by filling you without adding significant calories. Make sure you drink 4 to 6 glasses of water every day to assist the action of the bran in giving you proper bowel movements. You may find that you are a little "gassy" on a high-residue diet, but that will settle down after two or three weeks.

To get the maximum benefits from a high-residue diet, follow these suggestions:

1. Avoid refined simple sugars found in such foods as candy, soft drinks, breakfast cereals, and baked goods.
2. Avoid ultra-processed flour, usually found in white bread and cakes. Refined flour has practically no real food value.
3. Avoid all "junk" food.
4. Restrict beef and all fats, including dairy products.
5. Eat raw fruits and vegetables, with skins if possible.
6. Eat whole-grain products such as whole-grain cereals, unpolished rice and whole-wheat bread. "Instant" oatmeal and other "instant" cereals have been so refined that very little residue remains intact.
7. Drink 4 to 6 glasses of water every day.
8. Take 3 to 4 tablespoons of unprocessed bran every day at times that are convenient to you; the bran need not be taken all at the same time.

*Cholesterol, fat, and cancer** The Rechtschaffen Diet is a low-fat, low-cholesterol diet.

High-cholesterol foods include brains, egg yolk, kidney, liver, shellfish (shrimp, clams, oysters, mussels, lobster, crab), sweetbreads, dairy products and animal fat, including lard.

What is the difference between cholesterol and blood fats? Cholesterol is only one ingredient of blood fats. Cholesterol is found in such foods as milk products and animal fat (including butter).

Fish, chicken and veal contain acceptable levels of cholesterol. Egg whites, vegetables, fruits, whole-grains and cereals do not contain *any* cholesterol.

High-fat foods include fatty beef, pork and lamb; frankfurters; cake frosting; pies; butter and margarine; mayonnaise; and cooking fats and some oils.

Many foods contain practically no fat. A few of these are low-fat milk; most fruits and vegetables, including potatoes; light rye bread; and cooked rice and pasta.

I recommend that your daily food intake contain no more than 30 percent fat. Statistically a high-fat, high-cholesterol diet seems to be associated with cancer. Although few scientists are prepared to say *how* such a diet helps cause cancer, there have been some postulations made, especially in relation to breast and prostate cancer.

FAT CONTENT OF VARIOUS FOODS

Food	Size of Average Serving	Fat (grams)
Ground beef, broiled	3 ounces	17
Oils, salad and cooking	1 tablespoon	14
Pie, apple	1 piece (⅛ pie)	13
Butter	1 tablespoon	12
Margarine	1 tablespoon	12
Mayonnaise	1 tablespoon	11
Cheese, American	1 ounce	9
Liver, beef, fried	3 ounces	9
Bacon	2 slices	8
Milk, whole	1 cup	8
Potato chips	10 chips	8
Egg	1 large	6
Salmon, pink, canned	3 ounces	5
Pizza, cheese	1 piece (⅛ pizza)	4

FAT CONTENT OF VARIOUS FOODS *(cont'd)*

Food	Size of Average Serving	Fat (grams)
Yogurt, from low-fat milk, with added milk solids	1 cup	4
Fish sticks	1 stick	3
Bread, white, enriched	1 slice	1
Milk, low-fat	1 cup	0
Peas, frozen	½ cup	0

From U.S. Department of Agriculture, 1977.

How the Rechtschaffen Diet
Helps Lower the Risk of Heart Disease

Food Residue and Heart Disease   Even more than cancer, heart disease has been linked to diet. Heart disease in
America is responsible for more deaths than all other causes
combined.

During the past few decades the Ameican diet has changed
to include more animal protein, especially beef. Such a diet
means a large increase in saturated fats and cholesterol, both
of which have been implicated in heart disease. If saturated fats
and cholesterol are allowed to accumulate they can stick to the
inner walls of your arteries, narrowing the space for the passage
of blood. Also, the elasticity of the arteries begins to disappear.

Such a condition is known as atherosclerosis. It is dangerous because it cuts down blood flow, and if the artery is
closed off entirely, no blood flows through at all. If the closed
artery is in the heart, a heart attack occurs.* If the artery
takes blood to certain parts of the brain, a stroke occurs.

*There are other causes of a heart attack as well. For instance, we know now that a
heart attack may be caused by a spasm in the arteries of the heart.

A high-residue diet can help prevent the dangerous build-up of cholesterol in a very simple way. When you eat a high-residue diet, extra cholesterol is eliminated from your body along with your daily excretions. Cholesterol never gets a chance to accumulate, and one of the most serious causes of heart attacks is avoided.

Simple sugars and heart disease   The Rechtschaffen Diet is low in simple sugar for one obvious reason—simple sugars are fattening—but there are other reasons as well. A low amount of simple sugars in your diet will decrease free fatty acids in your blood, and will lessen the risk of heart disease.

The average American eats more than a hundred pounds of simple sugar a year. That's a lot of sugar. Just about every processed food contains sugar, usually more than we would guess—the amounts are rarely printed on the labels.

When you eat simple sugar you cause an increase of fatty acids (triglycerides) in your blood. Triglycerides combine with your normal blood glycerol to form the same kinds of fat as animal fat—*the same fats that we have repeatedly asked you to avoid.*

Not very long ago I had a patient who, when she first consulted me, had one of the highest triglyceride levels I had ever seen. It was 762, compared to the recommended level of 100 to 110! When she started my diet this woman weighed 220 pounds. Within four months she lost 40 pounds and her triglyceride level dropped to 354. Two months later she was still losing weight, and her triglyceride level was normal.

Salt and heart disease   If your physician can control the amount of salt in your diet, he can probably control your blood pressure. More than that, he can probably reverse your blood pressure if it is too high. *Usually atherosclerosis and hypertension (high blood pressure) are both reversible through diet.*

About 25 million Americans suffer from hypertension. It is sometimes called "the silent disease" because usually it is already a problem before it gives any indication that it even exists. Before you know it, a heart attack or cerebral hemorrhage can strike. The only real way to detect hypertension early is to have regular checkups that include a check on your blood pressure.*

When it comes to hypertension, salt and stress are probably your body's worst enemies.

In his *New York Times* column entitled "Knocking Salt Off Its Pedestal: Abstinence Without Remorse," Craig Claiborne wrote about his own love for salt. "For as long as I can remember," he said, "I could sit down to a plate full of anchovies with only olive oil, lemon juice or vinegar to dress it, and have a feast. A single salty sour pickle has never been enough for me. I prefer margaritas to other cocktails because of the rim of salt on the glass. Years ago in Japan I learned the pleasure of foods dipped in soy sauce (almost 100 percent salt) and lime juice. I have at times drunk that potion straight. A platter of salty, sour sauerkraut can almost be my undoing, and I have a craving for straight sauerkraut juice over ice."

He goes on. "A few weeks ago, I felt some disorientation while strolling down 57th Street. My balance was off and the sun suddenly seemed unbearably bright. An acquaintance familiar with my bizarre appetite for salt suggested I might be suffering from hypertension."

Fortunately for Mr. Claiborne, he was able to recognize

---

*It is a myth that your blood pressure is normal if it equals your age plus 100. In most cases such a number would be too high.

some early and tangible symptoms of hypertension, and he decided to seek a medical opinion. He came to my office, and I confirmed his hypertension. Now he eats almost no salt; his hypertension will probably remain under control as long as he continues to refrain from using salt.

Why does salt increase blood pressure?

Salt in your blood naturally attracts and retains fluid. This increases the amount of blood in your vessels at any given time. Salt also causes hormonal changes that may reduce the size of the opening in the arteries. If the same amount of blood is to be pumped to all parts of your body, the pressure must be increased to keep the blood moving through the smaller opening.

If you eat a lot of salt you probably find that you feel the need to drink a lot too. It's not just the salty taste in your mouth that's making you thirsty. Your body is telling you to drink more liquid in an effort to dilute the salt until you can finally eliminate it in your urine.

In cultures where no salt is used, people do not have hypertension, and blood pressure does not increase with age as it does in this country. In contrast, American children of parents who die before fifty of heart disease are likely to show early signs of problems of their own. The chances of high blood fat in these young children can be as high as 50 percent. The normal probability is one half of one percent—*100 times less.*

But even if you don't inherit a tendency toward heart disease, you may still be setting up problems early in life. Children who eat snacks containing large amounts of sugar and salt may be conditioned for future cases of hypertension and other forms of heart disease. This situation is aggravated by too little physical activity—a new trend for our children.

It's bad enough that children are snacking on high-salt,

high-calorie junk food, but they are doing it while *sitting* for hours in front of a television set.

⤦ Some High-Salt (High-Sodium) Foods

Anchovies	Monosodium glutamate
Antacids	Mustard (low-salt mustard
Bacon	is available)
Baking soda	Olives
(sodium bicarbonate)	Onion salt
Bouillon cubes	Pastrami
Canned soups, vegetables	Pickles
Caviar	Pizza (frozen)
Celery, celery salt	Pudding mixes
Cheeses (processed)	Relish
Chili sauce	Salad dressing (bottled)
Chipped beef	Salt pork
Cod (dried)	Salted and smoked fish, meat
Corned beef	Sardines (water-packed, no-
Cottage cheese (regular)	salt-added sardines are
Frankfurters	available)
Garlic salt	Sauerkraut
Ham	Sausages
Herring	Soy sauce
Ketchup	Table salt
Luncheon meats (salami,	TV dinners
bologna, etc.)	Worcestershire sauce (low-
Meat sauces	salt Worcestershire
Meat tenderizers	sauce is available)

Physical activity and heart disease   Regular physical activity helps your heart and blood vessels to work at peak efficiency. It increases the amount of oxygen transported from your blood to your brain and all the tissues in your body; it also increases the amount of oxygen your body can use.

When your muscles and other organs are receiving as much oxygen as they should, they will be ready to perform as well as possible when the demand arises.

Exercise helps keep your blood pressure under control by reducing the build-up of cholesterol and plaque on the inner walls of your blood vessels. It assists in keeping your blood fats at a reasonable level and prevents your blood from clotting too easily, and thereby blocking the normal flow of blood through blood vessels.

Finally, if you do have a heart attack, you will probably have a better chance of survival if you have exercised regularly.

To learn more about the benefits of physical activity see Chapter 4 on page 43.

Moderate drinking and heart disease   In 1974 the United States government published its *Second Report on Alcohol and Health.* The report raised some eyebrows by stating that moderate drinkers will probably live longer than people who do not drink at all. Rather than being harmful to the body, it has been found that *moderate* drinking may actually help prevent heart attacks. "Moderate" means 1 or 2 ounces of liquor or 4 to 8 ounces of dry wine consumed each day. No more.

High-density lipoprotein (HDL) is a fatty substance in the blood that seems to reduce the risk of heart attacks. Recently it was found that the blood of moderate drinkers usually contains a high proportion of HDL. In contrast, low-density lipoprotein (LDL) seems to be present in the blood of high-risk heart patients.* Smaller amounts of LDL are usually present in the blood of moderate drinkers. Based on this evidence, it seems likely that moderate drinking—and remember, this is strictly defined above—is at least one of the factors in reducing the risk of heart attacks.

Beer is a limited beverage because it is slightly higher in calories than wine and it contains salt, which remains in the bloodstream as a residue. After the first month on the diet an occasional glass of beer is permitted. If the taste of light, calorie-reduced beer is acceptable to you, drink it instead of the regular beers.

The use of alcohol *in moderation* almost certainly has real benefits for your body and your mind, but the abuse and over-use of alcohol will just as certainly lead to serious health problems, including cirrhosis of the liver. And of course, anyone taking drugs of any kind is cautioned about the possibly danger-ous combination of drugs and alcohol. If you are taking drugs, whether prescribed or not, consult your physician about the effect of alcohol.

Obesity and heart disease   Extra weight—even only 15 to 20 percent—will almost certainly increase your risk of develop-ing some form of heart disease, especially if you are over forty. In fact, if you are overweight, you almost double your chances of dying from a heart attack. (If you have diabetes and are

---

*HDL removes excessive cholesterol from body tissues, including artery walls; the cholesterol is then carried to the liver and excreted. Just the opposite happens with LDL, which carries cholesterol *from* the liver *to* the tissues. Some cholesterol is needed to help make bile salts, certain hormones and cell membranes, but excessive cholesterol is also carried to tissues. Lean people have higher levels of HDL in their blood than overweight people do. HDL is also found in relative abundance in nonsmokers, women and physically active people.

overweight—a frequent combination—you have increased the risk of dying of diabetes by almost *400 percent* above the norm.)

And the fatter you are, the worse off you are.

Your heart pumps blood throughout your body day and night without stopping for 70 or 80 years—that's about 100,-000 heartbeats a day, 2½ billion in a normal lifetime. Your heart was designed to do a job for a normal-weight person, not for a person 50 pounds overweight with high blood pressure and impending atherosclerosis.

Nutrition and Sex

An increase in sexual activity will not help you lose weight, but if you lose weight it may help you increase your sexual activity. Why?

It has been found that sexual intercourse is no more strenuous than taking a brisk walk around the block. In fact, it would take thirteen hours of sexual activity to lose one pound. So if you are looking for a useful exercise, try tennis or walking instead!

How are diet and sex related? In the first place, fat people just do not have the sex appeal of Robert Redford or Raquel Welch. Secondly, fat people usually have so much sugar in their blood that their sexual interest and performance are decreased. Crash diets almost always impair sexual potency, and may even create a psychological tension that makes it difficult to achieve sexual pleasure.

If the diet is adjusted so that blood fats are lowered, it is possible to prevent physical problems that cause impotence. Most of my diet patients tell me that *one of the fringe benefits*

of my diet and exercise program is that they have an increased ⌣
sexual desire and ability. It seems to be just a question of proper
maintenance—just the way a well-tuned car performs better
than a badly maintained one.

What about aphrodisiacs and Vitamin E?   Don't look for
"sexy" foods that suddenly turn you into a sexual athlete. No
such food exists. Most so-called aphrodisiacs are merely
sharp foods that irritate the urogenital tract. Such irritants,
whether they are foods or drugs, are potentially harmful, and
they certainly are not recommended. The closest thing I ever
found to a real sexual stimulant is a sensible program of a
well-balanced, low-salt, low-sugar, low-fat diet, exercise and a
relaxed attitude.

Some vitamins, especially E, have also been publicized
recently as enhancers of sexual vitality. Vitamin E dilates (en-
larges) the blood vessels, and in this way allows a free flow of
blood which increases the oxygen supply and produces a vigorous state. Exercise has the same effect, and is a lot more
reliable, especially because we are not fully able to predict the
possible side effects of massive doses of Vitamin E.

Getting Control of Your Life:
Some Fringe Benefits

Some joggers will tell you that they have a feeling of exhilara-
tion after a good run. Patients on the Rechtschaffen Diet have
told me they feel the same way after being on the diet for a
week or so. *There is a general feeling of fitness and well-being* ⌣
that comes from living on this program.

Much of this new feeling comes from a simple but immensely important change in your life: Your body is now functioning the way it is supposed to. You are *supposed* to feel this good! You are *supposed* to be in control of your life.

When your life begins to turn around for you it is exciting and liberating. You begin to look at the positive side again, knowing that things will go your way because you will *make* them go your way. One good experience leads to another.

One of my patients originally came to my office with a physical problem unrelated to diet. After we eliminated that problem we talked about the diet. She was slightly overweight, certainly not obese, but something told me that she would benefit both physically and mentally if she changed her lifestyle altogether. She resisted at first, but after a couple of weeks of complaining about having to change her eating habits she eventually decided to give the diet a fair try.

In less than two months she was feeling better than she had for many years. Even her arthritis had disappeared. Friends agreed that she looked younger and acted happier and livelier. She felt so good, in fact, that she started looking at her life for ways to make it even better.

She stopped smoking *because she wanted to,* not because anyone *told* her to. Now she takes pleasure in telling her story and suggesting that maybe you can want to make things better in *your* life.

It's an interesting idea, and I support it wholeheartedly. You will succeed with the Rechtschaffen Diet because you *want* to, and you will find new ways to make your life better too. You will be in control of your life. It has to be.

Chapter 4

The Importance of Exercise

Very often, when professional athletes retire they put on weight because, though they continue to eat the way they always did, they no longer exercise regularly. You may not be an ex-football player, but the same fundamental principle applies to you anyway: Regular exercise will help you lose weight or maintain the weight that suits you best. Without some physical activity you will probably have trouble using up all the calories you eat. What you don't burn off is turned into fat.

Regular exercise has other benefits. It makes you feel better. As we have seen, it also helps lower the risk of heart disease and other physical problems.

Exercise and Your Diet

Some of your friends will tell you that if you exercise you can lose weight without cutting down on fats and sugars. Others will claim that exercise is unnecessary if you watch your calories. Both are incorrect. There is no sense looking for shortcuts. If you want to lose weight *permanently*, you must follow a sensible diet plan *and* exercise regularly.

When you eat, you take in calories. When you are active, you burn up calories. If you take in more calories than you burn up, you gain weight. It really is that simple. That is why any permanent diet program must recommend that you exercise.

If you walk up a flight of stairs only occasionally, or if you start an exercise program on Monday and give it up on Wednesday, you won't see any change in your body. But when you exercise regularly (and that could mean walking; you don't have to become an Olympic track star) your body receives a message that something new is going on. Your built-in regulator begins to prepare your body for physical activity by burning off some excess fat. If your activity continues on a regular basis, and you also cut back on calories, you lose weight.

Before you do anything about strenuously increasing your physical activity, check with your physician.

Most people I talk with think that exercise increases your appetite. It doesn't. Exercise *decreases* your appetitie.

Exercise and the Circulatory System

Your circulatory system is made up of your heart and a complex network of blood vessels. All types of vessels—veins, arteries and capillaries—are important, but arteries are especially important because they carry oxygen-rich blood to all parts of your body.

We know that exercise can help prevent strokes and related problems. It appears that we increase our chances of a heart attack when we use less than 2000 calories a week in physical activity. This is not much exercise, certainly not too much for any of us to accomplish without a great inconvenience. If you were to jog three hours a week or walk six or seven hours a week you would use 2000 calories. Look at the chart below and see how your exercise routine fits in.

EXERCISE AND CALORIES

Activity	Approximate Calories Used			
	1 hr.	½ hr.	15 mins.	5 mins.
Walking* (slow; 2 mph)	150	75	38	13
Walking (medium; 3 mph)	300	150	75	25
Walking (fast; 5 mph)	480	240	120	40
Golf (with power cart)	200	100	50	17
Golf (carrying golf bag)	360	180	90	30
Typical housework	300	150	75	25
Scrubbing floors	360	180	90	30
Bowling	300	150	75	25
Bicycling† (slow; 6 mph)	300	150	75	25
Bicycling (medium; 8 mph)	400	200	100	33
Bicycling (fast; 12 mph)	600	300	150	50
Tennis (doubles)	360	180	90	30
Tennis (singles)	480	240	120	40
Ice skating/roller skating	420	210	105	35
Jogging (slow; 5 mph)	600	300	150	50
Jogging (medium-fast; 6+ mph)	700	350	175	58

*When you walk, 750 steps equal one-quarter mile; it takes 3000 steps to make a mile. *Brisk* walking is recommended.
†These figures also hold for an exercycle.

EXERCISE AND CALORIES *(cont'd)*

Activity	Approximate Calories Used			
	1 hr.	½ hr.	15 mins.	5 mins.
Skiing (downhill)	600	300	150	50
Skiing (cross country)	1200	600	300	100
Lawn mowing (with power mower)	250	125	63	21
Lawn mowing (with hand mower)	300	150	75	25
Swimming (medium)	400	200	100	33
Swimming (fast)	700	350	175	58
Gardening (light)	240	120	60	20
Gardening (heavy)	500	250	125	42
Wood chopping or sawing	500	250	125	42
Handball	550	275	138	46
Squash	600	300	150	50
Badminton	350	175	88	29
Disco dancing	600	300	150	50
Aerobic exercise	600	300	150	50
Hill climbing	500	250	125	42
Table tennis	360	180	90	30
Volleyball	350	175	88	29
Lying down or sleeping	80	40	20	7
Sitting	100	50	25	9
Driving a car	120	60	30	10
Standing	140	70	35	12

Exercise helps prevent circulatory diseases in many ways. It increases the efficiency of the heart and lungs, keeps the blood from clotting too easily, helps reduce the amount of fats in the blood, and helps prevent high blood pressure. If a heart attack does strike, it will probably be less severe in a well-conditioned person than in one who has remained sedentary.

It should be mentioned that people who smoke, have high blood pressure, or eat a high-fat diet increase the likelihood of a heart attack many times. Many heart specialists feel that the two greatest causes of heart disease are obesity and lack of exercise.

Other Benefits of Exercise

We are a people who want to be young, and at the same time we want to live to be a hundred. We look at those who have made it and ask why. What is the common factor that helps keep these centenarians alive and happy for so long? Excluding genetics, there seem to be *three* dominant factors common to elderly, vigorous people: 1) They are cheerful and emotionally stable; 2) They eat and drink in moderation; 3) They are physically active and like the work they do.

These three important elements in a full and happy life *are also the three most important elements in eradicating obesity.*

What seems to be the best and most common physical activity among people who live to be a hundred? Walking, according to a 1977 study by researchers from Europe, Canada and the United States, who reported their findings at a conference called "Exercise in Aging—Its Role in Prevention of Physical Decline." Even more than jogging, walking has been found to be the safest and most efficient form of exercise.

Your body was meant to be used. The less you use it, the less efficiently it will work. Although most of us may be doomed to creak and groan through old age, we can prolong the resiliency of our bones if we remain physically active.

There is new evidence that exercise may even help relieve diabetes and arthritis. Every day new research unfolds more benefits of exercise. If you are in good health, and your physician approves, exercise to feel healthier and younger. Your body is a remarkable machine. Use it or you'll lose it.

There seems to be little question that the benefits of exercise go beyond the physical. Usually, a person who is always tired will feel more alive and energetic after a few days of regular exercise. We know that physical activity improves oxygen transport to the brain.

The importance of exercise to counteract the effects of stress has been shown in a famous experiment by Hans Selye, one of the world's greatest authorities on stress. Selye subjected 10 sedentary rats to harsh lights, loud noises and electric shocks. Within a month all 10 rats were dead. Another group of 10 rats was subjected to the same stresses, but only *after* they had completed an exercise program. The exercised rats were still alive and healthy after one month of the same stresses that killed the sedentary rats.

We are not rats, but we probably respond to stress in a similar way. We all must find ways to soften the growing stresses of our modern age. Exercise will help.

How to Exercise Without Having
Your Own Swimming Pool

Some people don't have access to a squash court or a swimming pool. There are other ways to keep fit. If you want to exercise you can find a way that suits you. Take long vigorous walks. Walk six miles a day, in fact. Jump up and down. Jog in place. Walk up the stairs. Dance.

If you happen to be on the first floor of your home when you want to use the bathroom, use the one on the second floor. If the phone rings, get out of your chair and answer the extension phone at the other end of your house or apartment. Walk to the mailbox on the corner with your letters instead of having the mailman pick them up.

If you live on a low floor of an apartment house, walk up

instead of taking the elevator. And if you live on a high floor, take the elevator and get off two or three floors below your own. Get off the bus a few blocks before your stop. Instead of waiting for the bus to come, walk to another bus stop until it arrives. You will be amazed that even this much exercise can help you lose weight.

One of my patients and her husband decided to take a brisk walk every night after dinner. It must have helped, because after only a month they each had lost five pounds. (They also enjoyed the private time away from their three children.)

Park your car at the far end of the parking lot and walk to the market. Move around while you talk on the telephone. Train yourself to get up out of your chair—don't use your remote-control television channel changer, for instance, and move your wastepaper basket so you have to get up to reach it. Walk around every time a commercial appears on television. If you must watch television, ride an exercise bike or jog in place while doing it. And while you're at it, don't watch television so much. Most of us sit mindlessly in front of a television set for three hours a night because we tell ourselves that we're too tired to do anything else. The truth is, we're probably bored. Watch only the programs you really are looking forward to, and do something a little more stimulating with the rest of your time.

One of my patients puts on the original cast recording of *A Chorus Line* and lets nature take its course. Midway through the overture his entire family is bouncing around the house having a good time. I have found that listening to lively music while you exercise at home is an excellent way to avoid being bored. It also helps you exercise more effectively. Try it.

One of the nicest things about physical activity (it doesn't have to be "exercise") is that besides losing weight and looking better, you will feel better. After the initial period of adjustment you will breathe more easily, think more clearly and experience a feeling of muscle tone you haven't known since grade school.

Incidentally, you need not be concerned about taking salt tablets before, during or after strenuous exercise. Your food contains enough natural salt to replenish the salt you lose when you perspire. Too much salt during exercise can be a problem. Salt tablets taken before exercise can dehydrate your cells and cause nausea and muscle cramps.

In addition to walking about six miles a day (which is probably only about twice as much as you're walking now) or equivalent physical activity, you should also have thirty minutes of strenuous exercise at least three times a week. Such activity might be singles tennis, dancing, squash, brisk bicycling, swimming, handball, skating or just jumping up and down, jogging (even jogging in place) or walking up stairs.

Physical activity as strenuous as shoveling snow can literally kill you, especially if you are not used to working that hard. Don't push yourself to the point of exhaustion, and don't turn yourself against physical activity by overdoing it and hurting yourself. Unfortunately, some overweight people may overdo it on purpose just so that they will have an excuse for stopping. At that point they usually say something like "I'd rather be fat and alive than thin and dead." Well, I don't have to tell you that if you *are* fat you are probably shortening your life, so forget the excuses and be thin. Being thin doesn't have to mean being hungry, and that's what you're worried about most anyway.

Remember: Exercise does not have to mean dreary, tiresome, painful work. It means being physically active. It means using your muscles as they were intended to be used. It means using your arms and legs and *moving* your body. Don't sit when you can stand. Don't stand when you can walk. Don't walk if you can run. Move.

Chapter 5

The Rechtschaffen
Diet...
with Menus

You have probably learned that a diet is worthless unless it can be followed regularly, *without disrupting your entire life.* You also know that losing a few pounds (or even a hundred pounds) is meaningless if you sacrifice your mental or physical health. Of course, any decent diet must be based on an understanding of sensible nutrition.

The Rechtschaffen Diet is a permanent program of good eating that will help you lose weight if you wish, or help you maintain your present weight. *There are no foods you must stop eating forever.* The idea is simply this: Cut down on foods that are harmful to your body and concentrate on eating and drinking the foods that make you feel and look better. You not only do not give up your favorite foods, you will probably eat better than you ever have before.

Dieters have long known that the only diet they can really live with for any length of time is the one that can be varied according to what goes on in their daily lives. Also, a diet should not ask you to make an extreme change in your lifestyle. The Rechtschaffen Diet *does not ask you to count calories or to starve yourself.* It allows you to live normally—so normally, in fact, that you probably will not even think of yourself as being on a "diet."

The Rechtschaffen Diet meal plan is meant to be followed for four full weeks *without cheating.*

After you have achieved a realistic weight-loss goal for the first four weeks, you may begin to make occasional substitutions (such as beef, butter and shrimp). Your maintenance diet is outlined in Chapter 7—"After the First Month . . . Staying on the Diet."

Remember, the basic diet says:

1. Cut down on salt, simple sugars and fats.
2. Eat *more* complex carbohydrates.
3. Eat *more* high-residue foods.
4. Eat 3 to 4 tablespoons of unprocessed bran every day.
5. Drink 4 to 6 glasses of water every day, but *not* during meals.
6. Eat only 2 to 4 eggs every week, including those used in cooking.

THE RECHTSCHAFFEN DIET MEAL PLAN

1. The following menus have been developed for the first two weeks of the diet. Use them faithfully (but see item 2 below) without substitutions for two weeks and then repeat them for another two weeks until you have completed the first month. Then start the maintenance diet in Chapter 7.

2. Do not add to the menus or substitute anything—*except* that you may substitute for any dinner dish from the recipes that appear in the sections that begin on page 138; you may also substitute a veal, chicken or turkey dish for any fish dish. The dinner recipes will be especially useful if you have a little extra time or if you are having a dinner party.

3. Whole-grain foods include Wheatena, Farina, whole-grain oatmeal, pure shredded wheat, brown or white rice, grits, buckwheat or kasha, and couscous.

4. Whole-grain breads are made with unbleached flour. Some recommended breads are whole-wheat, sourdough and wheat-germ bread, unsalted whole-wheat Melba toast, pita and whole-wheat bran matzoh. All breads should be low-salt whenever possible.

5. Use only low-salt, low-fat cottage cheese, pot cheese and farmer's cheese. Some other popular cheeses like ricotta and mozzarella are now also available as low-salt, low-fat cheeses.

6. Coffee should be taken plain or with low-fat milk; tea should be taken plain, or with lemon or low-fat milk.

7. Eat chicken or turkey *without* skin.

8. Use only water-packed tuna fish, low-salt if possible.

9. Use only unprocessed bran.
10. You may have an alcoholic beverage with dinner if you wish. Choose *one* of the following: 4 to 8 ounces dry wine or 2 ounces scotch, rye, vodka or bourbon. Do not use gin or rum. Use all liquor straight or with tap water or low-salt mineral water or club soda only. If you prefer, you may have half of the allotted amount before dinner and half with dinner.
11. You may have your main meal of the day at lunch *or* dinner. Recommended dinner menus may be substituted at lunchtime (or vice-versa) if that is more convenient.

The menus follow, starting on page 55.

First Week

MONDAY

BREAKFAST

½ grapefruit
½ cup whole-grain cereal with plain yogurt or low-fat milk *Or* 1 slice whole-grain bread with low-salt, low-fat cheese
1 cup tea, coffee, decaffeinated coffee or low-fat milk

LUNCH

3½ ounces water-packed low-salt tuna with scallions, lemon and salad greens
2 slices whole-grain bread
1 cup tea, decaffeinated coffee or low-fat milk

DINNER*

Pineapple Watercress Cocktail (recipe on page 128)
Broiled fish
Parslied boiled potatoes
Tossed green salad
    French Dressing (page 173)
6 unsalted almonds or 6 unsalted filberts with a fresh fruit
1 cup tea, decaffeinated coffee or low-fat milk

*Veal, fish and chicken should be served in portions of 4 ounces, after cooking—more or less 6 ounces precooked.

TUESDAY

BREAKFAST

1 apple
½ cup whole-grain cereal with plain yogurt or low-fat milk *Or* 1 slice whole-grain bread with low-fat, low-salt cheese
1 cup tea, coffee, decaffeinated coffee or low-fat milk

LUNCH

4 ounces plain yogurt and 4 ounces low-fat, low-salt cottage cheese mixed with diced fresh scallions, cucumber, radishes and tomato, topped with freshly ground pepper if desired (page 165)
2 slices whole-grain bread or 1 board whole-wheat matzoh
1 cup tea, decaffeinated coffee or low-fat milk

DINNER

5 ounces no-salt-added tomato juice
Turkey Piccata (page 141)
Small baked potato
Hearts of lettuce salad
    Buttermilk Dressing (page 174)
Small banana or fresh peach
1 cup tea, decaffeinated coffee or low-fat milk

WEDNESDAY

BREAKFAST

1 wedge melon in season
1 egg, poached or cooked in Teflon pan
1 slice whole-grain bread
1 cup tea, coffee, decaffeinated coffee or low-fat milk

LUNCH

4 ounces broiled chicken
Lettuce and tomato with lemon
½ cup plain rice or 1 slice whole-grain bread
1 cup tea, decaffeinated coffee or low-fat milk

DINNER

Garden Soup (page 134)
Broiled Eggplant (page 166)
Tossed green salad
   French Dressing (page 173)
1 slice whole-grain bread
Navel orange
1 cup tea, decaffeinated coffee or low-fat milk

THURSDAY

BREAKFAST

½ cantaloupe or 5 ounces fresh orange juice

½ cup whole-grain cereal with plain yogurt or low-fat milk *Or* 1 slice whole-grain bread with low-fat, low-salt cheese

1 cup tea, coffee, decaffeinated coffee or low-fat milk

LUNCH

2 slices turkey

Mixed Vegetable Salad (page 178)

1 slice whole-grain bread

1 cup tea, decaffeinated coffee or low-fat milk

DINNER

Fillet of Sole with Almonds (page 149)

Small baked potato

Marinated Green Beans and Cherry Tomatoes (page 128)

Fresh pear

1 cup tea, decaffeinated coffee or low-fat milk

FRIDAY

BREAKFAST

½ cup fresh berries or 5 ounces fresh grapefruit juice
½ cup whole-grain cereal with plain yogurt or low-fat
  milk *Or* 1 slice whole-grain bread with low-fat, low-salt
  cheese
1 cup tea, coffee, decaffeinated coffee or low-fat milk

LUNCH

8 ounces plain yogurt mixed with fresh fruit
2 slices whole-grain bread
1 cup tea, decaffeinated coffee or low-fat milk

DINNER

Onion Soup (page 133)
Linguine or Spaghetti with Broccoli (page 157)
Watercress salad
  French Dressing (page 173)
Small fresh fruit cup without cherries or grapes
1 cup tea, decaffeinated coffee or low-fat milk

SATURDAY

BREAKFAST

½ grapefruit

½ cup whole-grain cereal with plain yogurt or low-fat milk *Or* 1 slice whole-grain bread with low-fat, low-salt cheese

1 cup tea, coffee, decaffeinated coffee or low-fat milk

LUNCH

4 ounces broiled fish

1 small baked potato

Sliced tomato

1 cup tea, decaffeinated coffee or low-fat milk

DINNER

Green salad with oil and vinegar

Veal Chop in White Wine Sauce (sauce optional) (page 144)

Brown rice

Shredded Zucchini (page 168)

Raw Applesauce (page 188)

1 cup tea, decaffeinated coffee or low-fat milk

SUNDAY

BREAKFAST

1 pear or other fresh fruit in season
1 egg, poached or cooked in Teflon pan
1 slice whole-grain bread
1 cup tea, coffee, decaffeinated coffee or low-fat milk

LUNCH

½ cup Spaghetti with Marinara Sauce (page 155)
Sliced cucumbers with vinegar
1 cup tea, decaffeinated coffee or low-fat milk

DINNER

½ grapefruit
Roast chicken
Curried Green Peppers (page 168)
Baked Buckwheat (kasha) (page 163)
Fresh berries with yogurt and cinnamon
1 cup tea, decaffeinated coffee or low-fat milk

Second Week

MONDAY

BREAKFAST

½ grapefruit or 1 small orange
½ cup whole-grain cereal with plain yogurt or low-fat
milk *Or* 1 slice whole-grain bread with low-fat, low-salt
cheese
1 cup tea, coffee, decaffeinated coffee or low-fat milk

LUNCH

2 slices turkey
Tossed salad with oil, vinegar, ground pepper
1 slice whole-grain bread
1 cup tea, decaffeinated coffee or low-fat milk

DINNER

Sizzling Fish Platter with Vegetables (page 148)
½ cup boiled rice
Apple or pear
1 cup tea, decaffeinated coffee or low-fat milk

TUESDAY

BREAKFAST

5 ounces no-salt-added tomato juice

½ cup whole-grain cereal with plain yogurt or low-fat milk *Or* 1 slice whole-grain bread with low-fat, low-salt cheese

1 cup tea, coffee, decaffeinated coffee or low-fat milk

LUNCH

3½ ounces water-packed low-salt tuna with sliced tomato, sliced onion, lemon

2 slices whole-grain bread

1 cup tea, decaffeinated coffee or low-fat milk

DINNER

Spaghetti with Garlic and Oil (page 156)

Stewed Mixed Vegetables (page 166)

½ cantaloupe or honeydew wedge with lemon

1 cup tea, decaffeinated coffee or low-fat milk

WEDNESDAY

BREAKFAST

5 ounces fresh grapefruit or orange juice
½ cup whole-grain cereal with plain yogurt or low-fat
    milk *Or* 1 slice whole-grain bread with low-fat, low-salt
    cheese
1 cup tea, coffee, decaffeinated coffee or low-fat milk

LUNCH

Spinach and sliced-mushroom salad with oil, vinegar,
    ground pepper
2 slices whole-grain bread
1 fresh fruit
1 cup tea, decaffeinated coffee or low-fat milk

DINNER

Veal with Tarragon (page 147)
1 small baked potato
Cabbage and Cucumber Salad (page 180)
1 cup tea, decaffeinated coffee or low-fat milk

THURSDAY

BREAKFAST

½ cup fresh berries in season or apple
½ cup whole-grain cereal with plain yogurt or low-fat
    milk *Or* 1 slice whole-grain bread with low-fat, low-salt
    cheese
1 cup tea, coffee, decaffeinated coffee or low-fat milk

LUNCH

4 ounces plain yogurt and 4 ounces low-fat, low-salt cot-
    tage cheese mixed with diced fresh scallions, cucum-
    ber, radishes and tomato, topped with freshly ground
    pepper if desired (page 165)
2 slices whole-grain bread or 1 board whole-wheat mat-
    zoh
1 cup tea, decaffeinated coffee or low-fat milk

DINNER

Mushroom Polenta (page 161)
Southern Fried Chicken (page 138)
Sliced tomato and lettuce wedge with lemon or vinegar
½ grapefruit
1 cup tea, decaffeinated coffee or low-fat milk

FRIDAY

BREAKFAST

1 small banana

½ cup whole-grain cereal with plain yogurt or low-fat milk *Or* 1 slice whole-grain bread with low-fat, low-salt cheese

1 cup tea, coffee, decaffeinated coffee or low-fat milk

LUNCH

Fresh fruit platter (no cherries, grapes or watermelon) with ½ cup cottage cheese

2 slices whole-grain bread

1 cup tea, decaffeinated coffee, or low-fat milk

DINNER

Poached Fillet of Sole with Tomato Sauce (page 152)

Potatoes Paprika (page 167)

Sliced cucumber with oil and vinegar

1 cup tea, decaffeinated coffee or low-fat milk

SATURDAY

BREAKFAST

½ grapefruit or 1 orange

½ cup whole-grain cereal with plain yogurt or low-fat milk *Or* 1 slice whole-grain bread with low-fat, low-salt cheese

1 cup tea, coffee, decaffeinated coffee or low-fat milk

LUNCH

Barley Soup (page 135)

Tossed green salad
    French Dressing (page 173)

1 slice whole-grain bread

1 cup tea, decaffeinated coffee or low-fat milk

DINNER

Stuffed Mushrooms (page 129)

Broiled Rock Cornish Game Hen (page 139)

½ cup brown rice

Orange Mint Cocktail (page 186)

1 cup tea, decaffeinated coffee or low-fat milk

SUNDAY

BREAKFAST

5 ounces fresh orange juice
2 eggs poached, boiled or scrambled in Teflon pan
1 slice whole-grain bread with 1 tablespoon low-fat, low-salt cottage cheese
1 cup tea, coffee, decaffeinated coffee or low-fat milk

LUNCH

Tabooley salad (page 179)
1 slice whole-grain bread
1 cup tea, decaffeinated coffee or low-fat milk

DINNER

Chickpeas Rémoulade (page 130)
4 slices cold chicken or turkey with hearts of lettuce, cherry tomatoes, with Blender Mayonnaise (page 176)
1 slice whole-grain bread
Melon wedge
1 cup tea, decaffeinated coffee or low-fat milk

RECOMMENDED MAXIMUM PORTIONS

Meat: 4 ounces, cooked, without bone or fat
Fish: 4 ounces, cooked, without bone
Poultry: 4 ounces, cooked, without bone, fat or skin
Vegetables: ½ cup
Fruit: 1 whole fruit, except ½ grapefruit, ½ cantaloupe,
    wedge honeydew
Juice: 4–6 ounces
Low-fat milk: 1 cup (8 ounces)
Alcoholic beverage: wine, 8 ounces total (2 4-ounce glasses);
    liquor, 2 ounces
Bread: 1 or 2 slices
Cereal: ½ cup
Whole-grain: ½ cup
Pasta: ½ cup
Matzoh: ½–1 board
Vegetable oil: 1 tablespoon
Low-fat cottage cheese: ½ cup
Yogurt: ½ cup
Potato: small to medium

FOODS TO AVOID

Anchovies
Avocado
Beer and ale
Brazil, cashew
    and macadamia
    nuts
Butter
Cake
Candy
Catsup
Celery*
Cherries*
Chewing Gum
Coleslaw
Cold Cuts
Cookies
Cream
Currants
Custard
Dried Fruits (figs,
    dates, apricots,

prunes, pears)
Frankfurters
Gherkins
Grapes*
Hamburgers
High-sodium
    mineral water*
Honey
Ice Cream
Jams and jellies
Jell-O
Mayonnaise
    (except
    homemade
    recipe
    provided)
Molasses
Mustard (except
    salt-free
    mustard or
    mustard
    prepared at

home with
    mustard powder,
    water and spices)
Pastries
Pickles
Pies
Pork products
Prepared salad
    dressings
Pudding
Raisins
Salt
Sauerkraut
Sherbet
Smoked Fish
Soda (including
    tonic water,
    no-cal and diet
    drinks)*
Sugar
Watermelon
Whole milk

*It is obvious that most of these foods are to be avoided because they contain too much sugar, salt or fat. But what about celery, cherries, grapes, mineral water and diet soft drinks? Celery contains salt, cherries and grapes contain a lot of sugar, and diet soft drinks contain artificial sweeteners that may be carcinogenic (cancer-causing). Some mineral waters are relatively low in sodium, others are higher.

SOME IMPORTANT POINTS ABOUT
THE RECHTSCHAFFEN DIET

1. Drink 4 to 6 glasses of water every day, but preferably not at mealtime.
2. Take 3 to 4 tablespoons of unprocessed bran every day. You may want to sprinkle it on your salad, cereal or yogurt, or mix it in meat loaf or other foods. Some people prefer to take it with their morning juice or fruit.
3. Conform to the diet without cheating for the first four weeks. No food is prohibited totally after the first four weeks. (See Chapter 7.)
4. Eat slowly. The faster you eat, the more you will eat.
5. Wherever possible, use fresh food. If that is impossible, use low-salt frozen foods but not canned. Canned food usually contains large quantities of salt and sugar.
6. Avoid artificial flavoring and coloring wherever possible.
7. Do not use sugar in any form. Refined sugar is a curse of civilization. Honey and molasses are also simple sugars; they are almost as bad for you as regular table sugar.
8. Avoid white bread, even if it's labeled "enriched." You need residue in your diet, and white flour is processed to the point where most of the residue is removed.
9. When the Rechtschaffen menus and recipes call for oil, try to use safflower or corn oil.
10. The Rechtschaffen Diet permits you to eat many more kinds of foods than most other diets. Portions should be kept fairly small. Serve veal, chicken and fish in 4-ounce portions.
11. If you are a vegetarian you can use the Rechtschaffen Diet without any inconvenience. Just substitute for meat and

fish dishes from other foods in the recipe section, making sure to maintain a proper nutritional balance.

12. After a short time on the Rechtschaffen Diet you will begin to feel more alive and healthy. At that point you will start to think about doing other things to improve your health. For instance, you will probably want to stop smoking. *You will not gain weight if you stop smoking.* The only time people gain weight after they stop smoking is when they substitute food for cigarettes.

Chapter 6

How to Make
the Diet Work
for You

By varying the Rechtschaffen Diet according to your personal
needs, you don't ever have to give it up. What you are doing
is adopting a whole new lifestyle that works for *you*, one that
helps you clear away the cobwebs in your head at the same time
you are clearing away the inches from your waistline. Along
with the diet, you will be involved in a natural exercise program
that does not demand much more than walking a little more
than you do now.

Unlike a crash diet, the Rechtschaffen Diet not only takes
effect quickly, it *remains effective* without harming the dieter.
Weight loss is slow and steady, tapering off at the natural level
your own body determines. The diet is based on the latest
nutritional research and recognizes the connection between
the foods people eat and the diseases they develop.

The Rechtschaffen Diet should be followed strictly for the
first four weeks—it may then be modified as needed. What is
important is that you try not to change the *quality* of the food

outlined in the Rechtschaffen Diet. Do not substitute foods that are not recommended.

If the Rechtschaffen Diet is followed even *most* of the time, you will feel both lighter and brighter. You stay on the Rechtschaffen Diet because you feel comfortable with it, and because it allows you to eat so well and to live so well.

Low-Salt Dieting and the Real World

I hope that one of the attractive features of the diet is its flexibility and understanding of how things are in the real world, *your* real world. No one can keep to a diet *all* the time. If you are in a special situation where you honestly feel like having a whole bottle of wine, go ahead. Enjoy it. You probably won't want *any* alcohol for a while. If your host and hostess have already salted the food, don't worry about it. Have your meal and enjoy it without feeling guilty. (Whenever you stray from the diet temporarily, no matter what the reason, don't feel guilty or doomed to failure. You will make up for it because you won't want those "forbidden" foods anyway.)

After you have been on the diet for a little while, you will realize that salt only disguises the true flavor of food anyway. Food actually tastes better without salt. Through the years your palate has been conditioned to accept salt, but after about three weeks without salt your taste buds will be fully acclimated to eating without salt—and you will taste the *real* flavor of your food for the first time in a long while.

If you eat kosher food your meat will be presalted. Wash the meat with cold water thoroughly before you cook it. The meat will still be kosher and you will have removed most of the salt.

Craig Claiborne, the eminent food writer of the *New York Times,* was not the most likely candidate to be on a low-salt diet. As we have seen, after being on the Rechtschaffen Diet for a few weeks, Mr. Claiborne was feeling and looking better than he had for many years. I had taken him off all medication and now he felt a clearheadedness and vigor that refreshed him every day. He lost 25 pounds and his blood pressure was normal after being dangerously high.

In an article he wrote for the *Times,* Mr. Claiborne described his happy experiences with his new diet. The article is too long to reproduce in its entirety, but here are two short paragraphs:

"Truth to tell," Mr. Claiborne writes, "I did not find strict adherence to a salt-free diet (with those rare departures) all that painful. Oddly enough, it was interesting, a kind of perverse test of character. I dined on more yogurt than I'd ever expected to take in my whole life. My consumption of tomatoes (another of my passions) exceeded its already large amounts. A cooked, unsalted tomato sauce became a daily accompaniment for fish, chicken, pasta, rice and potatoes (baked), cooked without salt, along with other foods.

"It would be the grossest deception," Mr. Claiborne goes on, "to pretend that salt-free cooking can equal the world's great cuisines. On the other hand, the food can be palatable and enjoyable. In my own case, my sense of taste seemed markedly sharper and, as time progressed, the various foods in the diet became more appealing."

Mr. Claiborne has told me more than once that he feels a renewed sense of enthusiasm and vitality, and he eats *more* than he did before. He is not my only patient who feels that way.

Your Food May Be Saltier Than You Think

Some high-sodium foods may not appear to be especially "salty," but all of the following foods contain high amounts of sodium: canned soup; packaged dinners, including TV dinners; canned franks and beans; bologna; canned green beans and most other canned vegetables; bottled pickles; antacids; fast-food hamburgers; prepared breakfast foods and chocolate shakes; processed cheese; instant beef broth; canned tuna; frozen pizza; regular cottage cheese; bottled salad dressing; instant pudding; and bacon.

Some foods that are not high in sodium become unacceptably high when they are processed and canned. For instance, fresh peas contain about 2 milligrams of sodium in a normal serving. The same size portion of canned peas contains approximately 100 times that amount of sodium.

It should not be your concern that manufacturers need to add salt to canned food to prevent spoilage or to "enhance" the flavor. We are lucky nowadays. When we can't get fresh food we can always get frozen food—that's still not the perfect solution, but by and large frozen foods contain less salt than canned foods do.

Adding Flavor Without Adding Salt

Most of my patients frown when I tell them to stop using salt. My food will be so *boring,* they say. Not so. Here are a few ways to spice your food without using salt in any form.

Try using a home-cooked, unsalted tomato sauce to add sparkle to such foods as veal, chicken or pasta. Become acquainted with scallions, shallots, leeks, garlic, onions and chives to enliven salads, sauces, soups, yogurt and meat and fish. Learn to make your own salt-free mustard from dry mustard powder, water and herbs if desired, and use it to add a sprightly flavor to meat and fish. Discover the unheralded world of fresh horseradish, delicious with cold salads or hot fish, or anything else you can think of.

Enjoy fresh fruit for meals and for between-meal treats. Bits of fresh fruit can be an appealing taste-enhancer when added to yogurt, cereal and other foods.

Experiment with pungent herbs, subtle herbs and exciting new herbs. The flavor of cooked food can be accentuated with a sprinkle of rosemary; tarragon; oregano; marjoram; a combination of basil, parsley, and oregano; salt-free mustard; turmeric; chervil; bay leaf; whole peppers; or a dash of paprika for color.

Pepper in its many forms, vinegar, and lemon or lime juice are other flavorful additions to a meal. Top off salads, oatmeal, rice and buttermilk, yogurt, cottage cheese and corn with freshly ground black pepper. Use vinegar and peppercorns on sautéed fish or veal. Squeeze lemon juice and sprinkle pepper on cauliflower or broccoli. Try crushed red pepper on eggplant spread, pasta, cauliflower, puréed vegetables such as broccoli and cauliflower, and on grated zucchini. Cayenne pepper is very hot, and should be used sparingly. Sprinkle a dab of cayenne powder on top of fish, veal, chicken and casseroles or stews. Incidentally, red and green peppers are excellent sources of Vitamin C.

A mixture of vinegar and dill makes a tingling topping for tomatoes and other fresh vegetables. Also, a dressing of lemon juice, vinegar and dill adds zest to plain broiled meat and fish or salads and fresh vegetables such as green beans, Brussels sprouts, potatoes and tomatoes. Vinegar or lemon juice are superb additions to almost any fresh vegetable.

If you use your imagination, you won't need salt.

Cooking with Wine

One way to cut down on salt (and to increase the flavor of your food without adding calories*) is to cook with a combination of wine, herbs, spices and succulent vegetables to create a flavor that goes beyond the capabilities of salt.

When you cook with wine you do not need to use an expensive wine—in fact, it would be wasteful. At the same time, do not use inferior wines that will contribute only poor taste to your food. Instead, use an inexpensive but reliable table wine whose label lists a reputable vintner and shipper. And by all means, do not use "cooking wines"—they contain a great deal of salt.

Your Diet and Your Budget

Some people say they cannot afford to buy exactly the foods they want. Usually you can get nutritious food that is on the Rechtschaffen Diet and is not expensive. Chicken, for example, is a great buy, as is turkey. Be careful not to go too far in economizing. I know a woman who said she could only afford to buy the supermarket "specials." Unfortunately, many of

---

*Doesn't cooking with wine add all the calories of the alcohol? No. An especially welcome feature of cooking with wine is that the alcohol in the wine burns off during cooking (eliminating the calories in the wine altogether), but the enriching flavor of the wine remains.

those low-priced items contain high amounts of salt, sugar and fat. When I first met this woman she weighed 231 pounds. She went on the Rechtschaffen Diet and within two months she weighed 209. It was a good start. Then she lost her job and started buying the "specials." When I saw her again her weight had gone up to 218.

Supermarket specials are not always a problem, however. Veal has been as low as $2.09 a pound when the regular price was about $5 to $6 a pound.

If you become familiar with the usual prices of foods, you will recognize a real "special" when you see it. As inflation gets worse and worse, reading labels and understanding value gets more and more important.

Pasta, rice and matzoh are always relatively inexpensive, and so are soups and chicken dishes. It's a good idea to look for foods that are abundant in your part of the country. Grain and vegetables are plentiful in the Midwest, for instance, and fish can be inexpensive if you live near the ocean and buy fish that is caught close to your hometown.

Of course, you can also save a lot of money on what you don't buy. Butter and beef are just two expensive foods you will not buy very often if you follow the Rechtschaffen Diet.

Losing Weight Because You Want To

Much of what happens with your diet depends on how you feel about it. It's like anything else. There's an old saying that says, "Be careful what you want—you may get it." If you want failure, you'll probably get it. So why not want success? You'll probably get that too!

One of the major keys to a successful diet is motivation.

Why do you want to lose weight? How *badly* do you want to lose weight? Do you care enough to *keep* the weight off?

If you want your diet to work you *must* do your part. You're like an actor in a play—you *must perform* every day. You must be an active participant, and not simply a bystander who is looking for a magical solution. You will decide what you want your lifestyle to be, and then you will share in the shaping of that style. You will take part in an active venture to change the way you look at yourself and the world around you.

But let's face it—you can't do it alone. You need reinforcement and encouragement from your relatives and friends. At first they may make it difficult for you by putting food in front of you and telling you to start your diet tomorrow, but you can change that too.

Once the people around you begin to understand that you mean it, they will respect your seriousness and do what they can to help you. And as you watch yourself succeed you will gain more and more confidence in your ability to live up to the principles of your diet.

Keep your mind open, especially to new ways of eating. Not long ago a woman came to me because she didn't seem to be able to lose weight. She said she had tried everything. We talked about exercise, food and her lifestyle in general. I made a specific suggestion about what she should have for lunch the next day. I recommended one of the handiest and least fattening dishes I could think of—diced radishes, cucumbers, scallions and pimentos topped with a heaping tablespoon of low-fat cottage cheese and a heaping tablespoon of plain natural yogurt. I suggested a sprinkling of freshly ground black pepper on top and then a gentle mixing so that the bright colors and different textures of the vegetables are distributed pleasantly throughout the cottage cheese and yogurt. Eaten with a couple of low-salt, low-sugar, whole-grain crackers or a piece of whole-grain bread, this dish is a favorite of mine and my patients.

My new patient wrinkled up her nose and declared that she hated yogurt. I suspected that she was not as sure of this as she seemed. I asked, "Have you ever tried it?" Without any feeling that it would make the slightest difference, she answered, "No." And yet she was sure she hated it.

A closed mind to new solutions can only result in the continuation of old problems. By being adventurous about food you will find more new treats than you can possibly imagine now.

Nobody Loses Weight Instantly

Don't lose weight for your doctor's sake. Do it for yourself. Losing weight is a day-to-day affair that requires *your* diligence, not your doctor's. Your doctor, friends and relatives all can help, and indeed they should help, but the main responsibility is yours. And the rewards will be yours too. Set a realistic goal for yourself. Two pounds a week—the average weight loss on the Rechtschaffen Diet.

Remember that you have not gained all your unwanted weight in only two weeks, so *don't try to lose it in two weeks.* The important thing to understand is that the extra weight *can* be lost. It makes sense to lose weight slowly, and in the process to learn how to *keep* it off. Most diet experts agree that the only sensible diet is one that you will be able to live with permanently.

If you aim to lose ten pounds a week and don't make it (and the chances are you won't) you will have one more reason to be discouraged about your weight. Don't create negative experiences for yourself. Set up challenges that *can* be met, and then reap the rewards.

Food As a Reward or a Tranquilizer

As you know, food is often used as a reward or a tranquilizer —but it shouldn't be. It started when you were a baby and you cried. Your mother fed you. Then you brought home that very nice report card that made everybody so proud. You had an ice-cream cone with sprinkles on it. Years later, you finished some work that nobody else could handle. Your boss took you to lunch and insisted you have an extra cocktail and a chocolate éclair, the specialty of the house. Just yesterday, you figured out how to fix the drippy faucet and saved $50 on a plumbing bill. You celebrated with a sausage pizza.

Don't feel guilty—everybody does it—but if you think about it, and you really want to change the pattern of your life a little bit, you can. The next time you feel you deserve a reward, buy yourself a tie or a blouse or a new recording of a Mozart piano sonata. Go to a movie. Get a personalized license plate. Join a tennis club. But *don't* have a banana split.

To Snack or Not to Snack?

Of course you should stop eating fattening snacks, but what will you eat instead? Fruit? Raw vegetables? Nothing?

Some people can't seem to stop their habit of snacking between meals or while they are watching television. When something signals you to start eating, that signal is called a "food cue." A typical food cue is walking into a movie theater. Who among us can resist looking for the popcorn machine before the movie begins? The tinkle of the little bell that announces that the coffee wagon is here also tells you that you want a cheese Danish, even if you ate a hearty breakfast just a short time before. You pass by a bakery on your way to the hardware store and you smell freshly baked apple pie. Who doesn't love the smell of freshly baked apple pie? You suddenly cannot live without a slice of hot apple pie.

You don't have to start nibbling just because you recognize one of your old food cues. Re-program yourself. Think of this: Who doesn't also love the smell of freshly cut grass? But you don't want to *eat* the grass, do you? You don't have to eat the apple pie either.

The next time you pass that bakery, enjoy the lovely aroma. But instead of going in and buying a pie, take a deep breath and give yourself a pat on the back for recognizing the cue for what it was: the signal to *smell* pie, not to *eat* it.

By the way, you don't have to sit through *Jaws III* or *The Godfather IV* without your popcorn. Order a *small* bag of popcorn, *without* butter or salt.

Some people have gotten into the habit of eating between meals because their families rarely sat down to a meal together. Many children get away with running in and grabbing a few mouthfuls between innings of a softball game. When these children grow up they probably won't care much about calm family dinners where everyone eats slowly and talks pleasantly.

Television trays should be banished from the house. How can a meal be important if you gulp it down in the living room during the evening news? Your dining area or dining room is what it says: a place for dining. Eat only in that place. Try not to eat in the kitchen. If you don't have a separate dining room, place a small table in your living room and put a festive tablecloth on it so that a definite part of the room is designated for dining.

Keep the Portions Small

I was recently told this story of what actually happened on a busy New York bus, where *anything* can happen. A very fat woman, about fifty years old, was sitting on one side of the aisle when a very trim woman, about twenty-five years old, got on the bus and took a seat on the opposite side of the aisle.

"Look at you," the fat woman said to the astonished young lady. "Look how skinny you are. I'll bet you're a model. Look at you. I eat an apple and gain two pounds. Look at *you*. You probably eat whatever you want and you *still* look like that. *Look* at you. My *cat* is fatter than you."

By this time, all heads were turned toward the object of all this attention. They wanted to know her secret too. The young lady squirmed in her seat for a minute, and then decided to assert herself.

"Listen," she said, "I go home and open up a can of soup, eat half and throw the other half away."

"What a waste!" gasped the fat woman.

"My refrigerator is a joke," the young lady went on, somewhat angrily. "I have a quart of low-fat milk, a couple of cucumbers, some cat food, and my cold cream jars in there. I buy something to eat on the way home. I *never* keep food around. You think I'd look like this if I kept food around? I'd be eating all the time, and I'd be just as fat as you are!"

Whatever you do, don't live the way this thin but unhappy young woman did. You can eat small portions of lots of good food without starving yourself. And don't be the fat woman who thinks it's a waste not to eat *everything*. You know she didn't really gain two pounds when she ate an apple. But she probably *did* gain two pounds when she ate a steak (with plenty of fat), buttered potatoes (large potatoes), creamed vegetables (two helpings), peach pie (two pieces) and, also, that apple.

Don't lie to yourself about how much—or how little—you eat. Follow the recommendations of the Rechtschaffen Diet, and do not think you have to lick your plate clean.

The Joy of Eating: Make Every Meal a Feast

Naturally, if you are on a diet you must know *what* to eat (or even more typically, what *not* to eat), but almost as important is the question of *how* to eat. The following suggestions will make your meals more pleasurable, healthier and more digestible:

1. Treat every meal as though it were a feast. Any food is more appealing if it is made to look attractive on your plate. Set your table as though you had guests. Colors and textures of foods are important. Add a radish to your salad or a sweet cherry pepper to a meat or fish dish to please your eye. The crispy texture of a chopped cucumber makes an interesting contrast with the smoothness of cottage cheese or yogurt.

2. Eat slowly and think about the taste of every mouthful of food. Not only will your food taste better, but you will lose more weight—food digested slowly will satisfy your hunger longer, and you will not be hungrily craving your next meal an hour after your previous one. End the meal with something bland; a bland food will not stimulate your taste buds and cause you to want a dessert.

3. Have no distractions at the dinner table. Concentrate on the task at hand. Never read or watch television during a

meal, even if you are alone; even a radio playing or people talking noisily can distract you from the full pleasure of your meal. A meal eaten on the run in the middle of midtown traffic does little good for your mind or body— and it will probably cause indigestion besides.

4. Make certain that every meal has more than one course, even if the extra course is only fresh fruit or tea. When the meal is finished you will feel satisfied without feeling full, and you will not be hungry until it is time for your next meal.

5. Encourage pleasant conversation at the table, but do not permit loud or harsh talk, or discussions of troublesome matters. Talk about the meal and think about the distinct taste of each food.

6. Feel free to eat dinner at different times; don't be rigidly locked into the habit of having dinner at the same time every night. The slight discomfort you may feel if you don't eat "on time" is strictly psychological; your body is perfectly able to wait an hour or two longer than usual. Don't overeat at the later hour to try to make up for the time waited.

7. In general, after the initial adjustment period of four weeks, you may deviate from the diet from time to time after you have attained your specific goals of lowering your weight and blood cholesterol (see the next chapter). This does not mean that you should feel free to gain weight and raise your blood pressure and cholesterol level. If you accept that piece of chocolate layer cake on Tuesday, try to be especially careful to trim off some extra calories on Wednesday or Thursday.

A final thought: Remember that you can stay on the Rechtschaffen Diet for the rest of your life without having to follow it totally. Except for the first month, when you should be as conscientious and thorough as possible in order to develop your own pattern and to learn discipline, you will be doing well to follow the diet about 90 percent of the time. And remember this also: *Don't feel guilty* when you do stray off the diet. There is probably nothing worse for the dieter than deep feelings of guilt (especially when those feelings lead directly to a large box of chocolates).

Relax. The Rechtschaffen Diet is meant for people who understand the joy of eating.

Some Useful Dieting Information

1. The faster you lose weight the more likely you are to regain it, because your usual eating patterns and long-term lifestyle have not been altered. Weight control requires effort, *and* a change of lifestyle.
2. If you eat only 100 extra calories a day, you will gain 10 pounds a year.
3. Avoid salt—it encourages the body to retain fluids, causing bloating and weight gain. This is especially true in women.
4. One large daily meal is more fattening than three or four small ones. This is true because when you eat a large meal your body secretes more digestive juices and you digest the food faster. As a result, you become hungry soon after a meal. Also, it is easier and healthier to digest smaller meals, and your body needs nourishment more than once a day. Some people like to eat more than three times a day. If you want to, you may take your total food allotment for one day and divide it up into four or five meals.

5. Physical activity (not necessarily "exercise") can alter the composition of your body, producing increased muscle and decreased fat. Decreased physical activity in later life invariably leads to increases of body fat, but middle-aged or older people do not *have* to get fat, as many of us are led to believe.

6. What you interpret as hunger may actually be something else—boredom, tiredness, depression, anger—even thirst. Very often you would be totally satisfied if you had a glass of water or juice—but you misread the signal and eat something instead. If you eat because you are depressed or tired, you will probably end up feeling even more depressed or tired. Keep active. *Boredom is one of the main causes of overeating.*

7. Don't eat to reward or punish yourself, or because you've had a bad day. Eat because eating is a necessary process that should be fun.

8. Many women abandon their diets because their faces tend to look thin before the rest of the body does. Your face will look natural again after a short time. Don't be discouraged when this initial facial weight loss prompts your friends to ask if you've been ill; in a very short time they will be asking you what you did to look so good.

9. When you lose weight, discard or quickly alter your clothes so you won't have your "fat clothes" to slip back into if you decide that dieting is not for you. Don't start dieting if you are only looking forward to stopping.

10. Buy small packages of food to avoid eating large quantities. Eat on small plates to reduce the size of your portions. Keep your portions fairly small, but not so small that you'll hate to look down at your plate. There should never be the need to cut thick slices of bread. A thin slice will do.

11. *Never shop for food when you are hungry.* Shop right after breakfast, but never just before dinner. If you shop for food when you are hungry, you will buy more food than you need—and once you buy the food you will eat it.

12. *Don't skip meals.* Eat breakfast *and* lunch so that you do not feel the desire to eat a large dinner and continue to snack afterward. It is especially important that you eat a good breakfast. If you seem to run out of time every morning, get up a little earlier—if you are older than thirty-five you don't need as much sleep as you used to anyway. (Don't sleep longer than you really need to. Your body uses more calories when you are awake than when you are asleep.)

14. Weigh yourself in the morning, always at the same time; but *don't weigh yourself every day.* You simply cannot expect to see the sort of results you would like on a day-to-day basis. If you are a woman you know that you accumulate fluid during the day; if you weigh yourself just before you go to bed, you will be at your heaviest, and you will have good reason to be discouraged. Avoid discouragement. Weigh yourself before your morning shower, and see the true benefits of your diet.

15. If you are going to cheat anyway, cheat with proteins and carbohydrates, not fats or simple sugars. If you are *really* starving, eat a little more of the foods I recommend, *not* the foods I ask you to try to avoid. Have a second helping of vegetables or chicken (without skin), but avoid the shellfish or ice cream except on infrequent occasions. But remember, you *can* do without cheating if you want to—you won't *really* starve, will you?

16. Eat slowly. The faster you eat, the more you will eat, and the sooner you will be hungry again.

17. Avoid sugar. Use cinnamon, pieces of apple, barley malt, nutmeg, or other fruits and spices instead of sugar.

18. If you are going to have a party on Saturday, don't buy the food for it on Tuesday—you may have eaten it by Thursday. Buy food when you need it—as close to the occasion as possible. For example, thousands of well-meaning dieters stock up on trick-or-treat goodies for Halloween ahead of time, and then eat them before the big day—when they have to restock again.

19. Don't *expect* a lapse into old habits. You *will* continue your new lifestyle even after you have lost weight.

20. *Don't create obvious temptations.* If you bake or buy a chocolate cake and leave it sitting on the kitchen table, you will naturally have a piece every time you pass by—and you may go out of your way to pass by.

21. *Act like you're thin already,* and you will get thin faster. Keep your shoulders back, hold in your midsection, and walk with a bounce in your step.

22. If you begin to gain weight, find out *why.* Then do something about it. Don't accept weight gain as unavoidable and inevitable.

23. Remember that *you are not alone.* About 50 million Americans are at least 10 pounds overweight. Most of my patients are not grossly overweight. On the average, they are about 15 percent heavier than they should be. So a man who comes to see me weighing 200 pounds should probably weigh 170, and a 140-pound woman would probably like to be 120 or 125 again. Those are not impossible goals. Don't feel sorry for yourself. You can lose weight permanently if you want to.

Chapter 7

After the First
Month . . .
Staying on the Diet

One of the most important points about the Rechtschaffen Diet is that there is no food you must stop eating forever. This is not a charitable act meant to impress you, nor is it a gimmick to lure you to try this diet. It is merely a sensible understanding of how people live.

If you have been on the Rechtschaffen Diet for four weeks you have probably lost 8 to 10 pounds by now. Also, you probably feel completely at ease with the diet—you don't want salt anymore, and you have survived well without beef.

After not having salt for four weeks your taste buds have changed. Your taste has actually become sharper. If you try salting your food again you will taste only the salt. It will be like eating pure salt. That's how your food *used* to taste. Now you can finally appreciate the taste of *food*, pure, fresh, unsullied food.

You may have noticed a subtle change that took place

three or four weeks after you started the Rechtschaffen Diet. You made a "mental switch" that changed your feeling about yourself and your diet. Instead of thinking about eating less, exercising more and losing weight, you suddenly became *part of your new way of life.* You didn't have to think about it anymore. You finally reached that point—a perfectly natural point—where your mind and your body come together and allow your body to function as it was designed to.

This sort of mental readiness sometimes occurs *before* a person begins a diet program. It's usually a sign that you are ready to make important changes in your life. Without your total acceptance of the idea of a *permanent* change you will undoubtedly continue to skip from one diet to another.

Your internal changes should be just as important to you as the obvious external changes—losing weight. In fact, you may find that losing weight is really a secondary process of a much more important change that reinforces your whole new way of life.

You may also find that you are able to eat more food than you did before the diet—*without gaining weight.* This will happen as long as you do not eat the high-salt, high-fat, high-simple-sugar, low-residue foods you are supposed to avoid. It is much worse to change the quality of your food than to change the quantity of recommended foods. You really can eat more and weigh less if you choose the proper foods.

You used to put things off until tomorrow—you don't anymore. Now you want to get things done as soon and as well as possible. You used to ignore your overall health—you don't anymore. Now you have come to realize that by maintaining your good health you don't have to think about treating disease anymore. Good health means *preventing* disease, not just treating it. The natural state of your body is to be healthy, not to be sick. It's one more aspect of your total positive approach—you will maintain your good health as well as your best weight.

By now you have developed a satisfaction in your ability to respond to discipline and change. You are also at ease no matter *where* you have dinner, mainly because your new confidence permits you to eat as *you* want to, no matter what other people say or do.

By now you are learning how to relax also. Relaxation is important in your general feeling of confidence and well-being. Unfortunately, it doesn't come easily in the midst of the daily tensions of your job, home, school and children. Nonetheless, you must relax and be at ease so that your clarity of thinking is not impaired by everyday problems and tensions. Even as the daily concerns and joys fluctuate up and down, you must learn to remain steady—on an even keel that is not affected by the artificial very high "highs" and the very low "lows."

Take a deep breath from way down in your abdomen and learn to breathe so that your diaphragm gets into the act as it is meant to. And when those highs or lows come along, tell yourself, "Relax, relax, relax."

You've come a long way, and you have a right to be proud. Now you want to make sure that nothing gets in your way of total success—you really *do* want to keep feeling and looking as good as you you. And you can.

You can keep going. There is no reason to slip or to become bored with the diet. In fact, this may be the most important phase of the diet. If you can continue to do as well as you have, you will have no trouble maintaining your new lifestyle forever. You owe yourself a treat. I also owe you something.

The Rechtschaffen Diet has promised that you may eat your favorite foods once in a while—no matter *how* many calories they contain. And it's true. You don't have to give up strawberry shortcake forever. Look at the following list and see how many new substitutions and allowances are acceptable now that you have established your new lifestyle.

After the First Month . . .

1. You may have a 4-ounce portion of cooked lean beef, lamb, pork or shellfish once a month.
2. You may increase the size of your portions (especially of bread) if you would like to *gain* weight. As incongruous as that sounds, many people do lose more weight than they thought they would, and they would like to put back a couple of pounds.
3. You may have a pat of butter once a week.
4. You may have a piece of fruit between meals.
5. You may have a glass (8 ounces) of beer with dinner or lunch once a week. "Light" beers are recommended because they contain fewer calories than regular beers do.
6. You may want to pick one day a week (Sunday is usually the favorite) when you make the exceptions and eat the foods that are permitted only occasionally.
7. You may dine out with friends without any diet restrictions once a month.
8. If you cheat after the first month (and I hope you won't), don't cheat with sweets. You will be much better off with occasional extra starches instead of simple sugars.
9. Remember that you are in control of your life. Never again will food have to become the one gratifying experience you crave.

AN OVERALL VIEW OF THE RECHTSCHAFFEN DIET

(Note that menus and recipes to implement this meal plan appear on pages 55 and 118. Recommended portions are specified in the menus, and a list of recommended maximum portions appears on page 69).

You may eat 2 to 4 eggs a week, including those in processed foods and cooking *if* your doctor approves your cholesterol level. Use a Teflon pan to eliminate the need to use butter or oil.

TO BE TAKEN DAILY:

1. 4–6 glasses of water
2. 3–4 tablespoons of unprocessed bran

BREAKFAST:

Fruit or juice

Whole-grain cereal with plain yogurt or low-fat milk
Or Whole-grain bread with low-salt, low-fat cheese

Tea, coffee, decaffeinated coffee or low-fat milk

LUNCH:

Yogurt with fresh vegetables or fruit
Or Meat, chicken, turkey or fish
Or Vegetable or fruit platter
Whole-grain bread or whole-grain food
Tea, decaffeinated coffee or low-fat milk

DINNER

Soup (occasionally)
Meat, fish, chicken, turkey or pasta
Salad
Whole-grain bread or whole-grain food
Fresh fruit
Tea, decaffeinated coffee or low-fat milk
Alcoholic beverage if desired

Chapter 8

Living Well on the Rechtschaffen Diet

Nothing can be more unsettling to a person on a diet than not to have control over what to eat. Your own home is safe, a familiar environment where you eat what and when you want. You are in charge. But what happens when you are invited to a friend's house for dinner or a party, especially a birthday party? And how can you possibly stay on your diet when you're having dinner at a restaurant? It's not as hard as you think.

Rehearsing for Restaurants

Before you go to a restaurant, think about what will happen once you get there. Even the thinnest person in the world would be tempted to order everything on the menu—you're *supposed* to be tempted. After all, restaurants don't make any money serving plain toast and black coffee.

Since you already know that the restaurant's menu is going

to be enticing, plan ahead and be prepared to take charge and make sensible choices. To start with, there's no reason not to have an hors d'oeuvre. Plan to select one that stays within the basic regimen of the Rechtschaffen Diet. For example, order a salad or melon. (When you order a salad ask the waiter to bring the oil and vinegar and put a light dressing on the salad yourself. Don't order the house dressing because it will contain salt.) While you're waiting for what you've chosen to arrive, do not sample those rolls. In fact, if you feel it is not appropriate to ask the waiter to remove the bread or rolls, at least make sure that they are placed in front of someone at the opposite side of the table.

When the time comes to order the main course, don't limit yourself to choosing from the menu if there's nothing there that fits into the Rechtschaffen Diet. Say, "I would like (whatever you would like). Can you make it?" Usually the head waiter will be happy to give you what you want. If he can't give you exactly what you asked for, he can probably prepare something just as suitable.

Don't worry about hurting the chef's feelings. When I first started to dine at what now is my favorite Chinese restaurant I asked for no salt, no monosodium glutamate, no soy sauce and lots of spice. The head waiter smiled and rushed off to the kitchen. When he came back with the food he was obviously pleased with it. He leaned close to my ear and said, still smiling, "Finally we can serve our food the way *we* eat it!"

Also, don't worry about appearing strange to your fellow diners when you make a special request. They won't be embarrassed; in fact they will respect you for it. They may even do the same thing the next time they go to a restaurant. As one of my friends said to me, "I didn't know you could make special requests." You can.

The Shun Lee Palace is one of New York City's finest restaurants. Co-owner Michael Tong enjoys the challenge of adapting his recipes to agree with the principles of the Rechtschaffen Diet; so do other fine restaurants all over the country. Here are two examples of Shun Lee recipes prepared without salt, sugar, animal fat or monosodium glutamate:

POACHED FLOUNDER WITH SCALLION SAUCE

1 flounder (about 1½–2 pounds)
10 cups water
2 tablespoons vegetable oil
2 tablespoons fresh ginger, shredded
4 cloves garlic, finely chopped
4 scallions, including green part, shredded into thin strips about 1½ inches long
2 tablespoons sherry

1. Bring water to a boil in wok or pot.
2. When water is boiling place flounder in it carefully. Cover.
3. After 2 minutes remove from heat. Allow fish to simmer in water about 5 minutes.
4. Remove flounder from water and place on plate.
5. Drain water from wok.
6. Heat vegetable oil in wok to 450°.
7. Sauté ginger, garlic, scallions and wine for 15 seconds. Pour over fish and serve.
   Yield: 4 servings

SLICED VEAL HUNAN STYLE

1 pound veal steak
6 cups water
15 slices water chestnuts
15 snow peas
2 tablespoons vegetable oil
½ tablespoon chopped garlic
3 tablespoons chopped scallions
1 teaspoon fresh ginger, shredded
½ teaspoon dry Szechuan pepper seeds or crushed red pepper
2 tablespoons dry sherry

1. Place veal steak on flat surface and cut into thin slices.
2. Bring water to a boil.
3. Cook veal slices in boiling water for 30 seconds. Add water chestnuts and snow peas for 10 additional seconds.
4. Drain veal and vegetables quickly in colander.
5. Heat vegetable oil in wok or frying pan to 450°.
6. Place garlic, green onions, ginger and Szechuan pepper seeds into vegetable oil, and cook for 10 seconds.
7. Add veal, snow peas, water chestnuts to wok and sauté entire mixture for 20 seconds.
8. Add sherry and serve.
   Yield: 4 servings

Dessert time is easy. Order fresh fruit, and don't give the pastry tray a second thought. Every waiter I have ever met thinks it's cute to lure you into having a dessert by making a big production out of wheeling the pastry cart as close to you as possible. He can see that look in your eye when you are weakening, and he won't give up until you order the largest, gooeyist thing on the tray.

Don't give the waiter a chance. When you order your entrée tell him you would like fresh fruit for dessert. If he says there is no fresh fruit tell him firmly that you do not want any dessert; just black coffee, thank you.

Waiters are not the only ones who will try to tempt you in restaurants. Until your friends realize that you are serious about your diet they will be just as cute as the waiter in trying to force a dessert on you. Just say, "No, thank you. The meal was so good I don't have room for another thing. But you go ahead anyway." Stick to your guns, and you may find that your friends skip dessert the next time too.

Restaurants usually serve large portions. You don't have to eat the whole thing. As usual, people are not watching you as closely as you think they are.

If you are having lunch or dinner at a restaurant, or if you are on a business trip, remember: Any good restaurant will be flexible enough to prepare variations of their dishes. Don't be afraid to ask.

How to Cope with Parties

It is all right to have a drink or two at a party. But there will be so many good things to nibble on that you should be prepared to make your nibbles count. Nowadays, most hostesses offer fresh uncooked vegetables and a dip of some kind, often with a cream cheese base. Eat the vegetables (except celery), but skip the dip.

Vegetables alone may get to be a little boring after a while, so pick something that seems especially appetizing to you and have *one*. Only one. The dieting problems at a party arise when you eat five or six tidbits that are not on the diet. But one won't hurt. Have a light lunch the next day to make up for it.

A wonderful way to work off some extra calories at a party is to dance. A few minutes of disco dancing will use up about 50 calories, and if you dance for half an hour you will use 300 calories, as much as in a cup of baked custard.

How to Go on Vacation
Without Ruining Your Diet

Vacations are important. They should be enjoyed as fully as possible, without the ordinary pressures and timetables. But this does not mean that you should use a vacation as an excuse to forget your diet entirely.

Vacations can be even more challenging than dining out or going to a party. To be realistic, you probably should not expect to lose weight while you're on vacation. Instead, try to maintain your weight.

One of my patients travels about one week out of every month. Before I met him he usually ate cereal, milk and fresh fruit for breakfast when he was at home. Sometimes he added toast and coffee. When he was out of town, however, he changed his breakfast routine altogether. Faced with a hotel menu, he invariably had juice, eggs, bacon, buttered toast, coffee and hash-brown potatoes. If he had time he would order extra toast and eat it with jelly. He didn't have a special reason for changing his breakfast pattern, but he did it every time. When his wife offered him the same things at home he wasn't interested.

Such behavior is typical of people on vacation. To a certain extent we all do it. After all, isn't a vacation a time for total fun and relaxation? Sure it is, but who says gaining weight is fun? *Eating* is fun. Gaining weight is boring.

Plan on straying a little bit while you're on vacation. Know ahead of time that you'll do it, and don't feel guilty when it happens. Cut back a little bit at breakfast and lunch. Swim or ski instead of lying in the sun or sitting in the lodge *all* the time. Walk and explore the new territory. Then have something really special for dinner. Keep the portions to a sensible size and don't have seconds.

If you follow the Rechtschaffen Diet *most* of the time and remember how important it is to be physically active, you will be surprised at how little weight you will gain on your vacation.

Incidentally, before you make your hotel reservation, check to make sure they will be able to adapt their menu to your diet.

Dieting on
an Expense Account

Expense account meals are different from other meals. Almost always, an expense account lunch is also a business meeting. Admittedly, you may be more concerned about pleasing your client than staying on your diet.

If ever you were in control of a meal, it's this one. Don't forget, *you're* paying the check. You have chosen the day, the time and the restaurant. Presumably it's a restaurant where you are fairly well known and where you know the menu. If it isn't, when you call for a reservation, find out what is on the menu for that day. You will usually find a fish, veal or chicken dish (and don't forget a medium-sized portion of pasta) that will be excellent for you.

There is no need to make your diet the central topic of conversation, but no harm will be done if you decline a dessert or a liqueur with a simple statement that these foods are not included in your diet.

If *you* are the guest at a business luncheon, you will have no trouble with your selections. Your host will be more concerned with pleasing you than whether or not you are having a chocolate éclair.

Don't forget a cardinal rule of the Rechtschaffen Diet: If you are in a situation where *no other alternative is possible,* go ahead and order the liqueur or steak. You don't have to finish it. In fact, you probably won't *want* to finish it.

There is another important choice you can make. If you know you are going to be eating a business lunch today, or even if you are just having lunch with a friend, make it your big meal of the day. Switch lunch and dinner. When you get home you can eat a salad for dinner or yogurt and cottage cheese with diced raw vegetables. Keep your meals flexible, and don't automatically make dinner your biggest meal of the day.

Birthday Parties and Dinner Parties

Have you ever made the mistake of declining a piece of cake at a birthday party? It's a sure way to look like a villain. Take the cake, but don't eat much of it. There is so much going on at a birthday party that you can easily put your plate down somewhere as you move off to check the presents or help pour the juice.

There is another social gaff you can make in the name of your diet. Have you ever been invited to someone else's house for dinner and then refused half of the meal because it wasn't "on your diet"? The same rules apply here as at a birthday party. There is no need to hurt your host's or hostess' feelings and call undue attention to yourself by making a fuss about the food. Your host and hostess have worked all day (maybe even longer) to plan and prepare the dinner. It is a special occasion for them. Don't spoil it.

Try to keep the portions small, or leave some food on your plate. You will be more gracious if you say you are too full to finish (if anyone notices) than if you don't eat anything at all. You can always plan your own menus around these special dinners so that you cut down a little bit the next day if you have to. In fact, *don't forget* to cut down a little bit the next day.

As you know, it's all too easy to accept permission to go off your diet for one day without doing anything to balance the off-day. The Rechtschaffen Diet is not a regimen of torture and deprivation, but neither is it a license to forget yourself completely.

Chapter 9

Questions People Ask About Dieting

Q. *Is fatness inherited?*

A. Not really. The *potential* to become fat may be inherited, but that does not mean you have to become fat. Usually fat parents feed their children too much and don't put enough emphasis on physical activity.

Q. *Are women necessarily fatter than men?*

A. Most women gain weight more easily than men do, and they have more trouble losing it. Nevertheless, this should not be taken to mean that women are destined to be fat.

Q. *Why is it that a person on a diet is permitted to eat baked and boiled potatoes but not French fries, home fries or mashed potatoes?*

A. Potatoes by themselves are not fattening, and boiled or baked potatoes are completely acceptable as long as no butter or cream is added. Baked sweet potatoes may also be eaten if nothing is added. The problems begin when we cook the potatoes in oil, for example, or when we add such ingredients as salt or butter. French fries are unacceptable because too much oil may be used and salt is invariably added; other fried variations are equally unacceptable for the same reasons. A typical serving of mashed potatoes contains butter and milk, and therefore is not encouraged, but try fixing mashed potatoes with yogurt, low-fat milk, pepper, dill, parsley and chopped onion or scallion instead.

Q. *Is putting on weight periodically all right as long as you keep taking it off?*

A. No, it isn't. When you continually put on weight and take it off you put more strain on your heart than if you gained a few pounds and left them on. Either don't gain weight in the first place, or if you do gain weight and want to lose it, lose it permanently.

Q. *Does the food you eat have anything to do with cancer?*

A. In 1979 the National Cancer Institute advised that the risk of cancer could be reduced by eating less and by eating a low-fat, high-residue diet.

Q. *Is the food you eat sometimes related to heart disease?*

A. Yes. Heart disease seems to be most prevalent when a diet is too high in fats, saturated fats, cholesterol and salt, and too low in polyunsaturated fats and carbohydrates.

Q. *Is it true that in order for any diet to be successful you cannot go off it, even for a day or two?*

A. No, that is not true. If a diet is to be realistic it must allow for a lapse *once in a while*. But if you go off your diet on Tuesday, you should reduce your food intake appropriately the next day. If you make a *habit* of going off your diet you certainly will be unsuccessful in losing weight.

Q. *Why is whole-grain bread favored over white bread?*
A. Whole-grain cereals and breads contain the residue needed to decrease the time it takes for food to pass through the large intestine—the longer the food remains in the large intestine, the greater is the chance of intestinal cancer. Also, by eating whole-grain breads, which are bulkier and heavier than white breads, you cut down the quantity of food you need to satisfy your hunger. White bread is merely "empty calories," with no minerals, no vitamins, and no nutritional value, and cake is loaded with harmful simple sugars. In contrast, whole-grain bread has many beneficial natural nutrients.

Q. *Isn't "enriched" white bread as healthy as any other bread?*
A. "Enriched" white bread is enriched with very little that will help you. Ordinarily, white bread contains sugar and salt, and has very little food value, if any.

Q. *Are all additives bad for you?*
A. No. In fact, some preservatives are necessary to curtail the action of harmful bacteria. As a rule, though, you should avoid artificial food coloring and flavoring and eat fresh food whenever possible.

Q. *Should you cook only with cooking wine?*
A. On the contrary, *do not* use cooking wine for cooking. It contains a great deal of salt, and is undrinkable. Use an inexpensive but reliable table wine instead.

Q. *Doesn't cooking with wine add calories to a meal?*

A. No. The alcohol in the wine burns off during cooking, eliminating the calories in the wine altogether.

Q. *If you are on a diet can you ever drink beer?*

A. It's not a good idea to drink beer during the initial adjustment period of 4 weeks, but once you have lost about 8 to 10 pounds, you can have a beer occasionally.

Q. *Why are gin, rum and liqueurs not allowed?*

A. Gin is made from the juice of the juniper berry, which has an adverse effect on the central nervous system and seems to cause rapid intoxication; rum contains many calories because it is made with cane sugar; liqueurs have a very high sugar content.

Q. *If you drink a lot of water won't you get bloated?*

A. No. You should drink 4 to 6 glasses of water every day. Bloating usually occurs just before a menstrual period or if you eat too much salt.

Q. *If you eat beef should you buy only the best cuts?*

A. Not necessarily. The less expensive cuts, like flank steak, usually contain less fat than the expensive cuts.

Q. *Aren't two eggs every morning the basis of a healthy breakfast?*

A. No. Egg yolks contain a high amount of cholesterol, and egg whites are high in sodium. You should eat no more than 2 to 4 eggs a week, including those in cooking and processed foods.

Q. *Is celery a good diet food?*

A. No. It contains too much salt.

Q. *Is flavored gelatine a good diet food?*

A. No. It contains too much simple sugar or, in the case of sugarless products, contains artificial sweeteners which may be dangerous.

Q. *Is chewing gum a good distraction from food?*

A. No. It contains too much sugar, and sugarless gum contains artificial sweeteners which may be harmful.

Q. *Can dieters ever eat potato salad?*

A. A small portion of potato salad is all right if it is made with homemade mayonnaise that does not contain salt and sugar.

Q. *Is an apéritif before dinner good for your digestion?*

A. Perhaps, but most apéritifs add calories to your meal and cause you to eat more by stimulating your appetite.

Q. *Will you gain weight if you stop smoking?*

A. No. People only gain weight when they stop smoking if they substitute food for cigarettes.

Q. *Should you drink plenty of water with your meals?*

A. No. Too much water *with* meals dulls your taste buds and dilutes your digestive juices. No more than one glass of water should be had with a meal, and it should be sipped slowly.

Q. *Should you always eat your meals at the same time each day?*

A. Not necessarily. It would be more realistic to be flexible about it.

Q. *Should you feel guilty when you "cheat" on your diet so you won't do it again?*

A. No. Don't feel guilty, but do try to make up for the lapse the next day by eating less.

Q. *Isn't hamburger an almost perfect food?*

A. Definitely not. Hamburger contains a great deal of fat, and fast-food hamburgers usually contain quite a bit of sugar to make them brown quickly, salt, and other objectionable dressings or relishes. Besides, a hamburger is made of beef, which should be strictly limited on your diet.

Q. *Is popcorn fattening?*

A. By itself popcorn is not fattening. It becomes fattening when you add salt and butter.

Q. *Are people born with a taste for salt?*

A. No. The taste for salt is an acquired one.

Q. *For a diet to be successful, must you lose weight quickly?*

A. On the contrary, a slow and steady weight loss is characteristic of a diet that keeps the pounds off permanently.

Q. *Can diet pills hurt you?*

A. Some diet pills can aggravate cases of high blood pressure and other heart-related diseases, diabetes, and thyroid disease. Other types of diet pills may cause nausea and dizziness and may even upset your hormonal balance.

Q. *Are all diets recommended by doctors nutritionally sound?*

A. Unfortunately, no.

Q. *Are all Americans well nourished?*

A. No. Just because you are not hungry, underweight or overweight does not necessarily mean you are following a healthy, well-balanced diet. About half of the American population eats too much "junk" food.

Q. *Do baby foods need salt and sugar to please the baby?*
A. Salt and sugar are put into baby foods to please the mother, not the baby. Some baby-food companies no longer add salt and sugar, with no loss of sales.

Q. *Will an extra 100 calories a day add weight?*
A. Yes, about 10 pounds a year.

Q. *Are you destined to be overweight once you reach middle age?*
A. Not necessarily. If you watch your diet and keep physically active you should not gain weight.

Q. *Should food be used as a reward?*
A. Food should never be used as a reward, and sweets are terrible for children *or* adults. Sugar is bad for you, and should not be referred to as a "treat."

Q. *Is all sugar the same?*
A. There are two types of sugar: complex and simple. All types of table sugar are simple sugars, and are not recommended.

Q. *Won't I be better off using honey or molasses instead of sugar?*
A. No. Honey and molasses both contain simple sugars, which makes them the same as ordinary sugar. In addition, honey and molasses contain more calories than sugar does.

Q. *Is brown sugar more nutritious than white sugar?*
A. No. The color of brown sugar is caused by impurities. Both brown and white sugar are simple sugars, and are not recommended for regular use.

Q. *Has the United States government made any recommendations about our diets?*

A. In February 1980 the United States government took a historic step by issuing a formal recommendation for good nutrition. It recommended that we eat a variety of foods; maintain ideal weight; avoid too much fat, saturated fat and cholesterol; eat foods with adequate starch and residue; avoid too much sugar; avoid too much salt; drink alcohol only in moderation. The Rechtschaffen Diet makes the same recommendations.

Q. *If you reduce your calorie intake, will you lose weight automatically?*

A. No. Decreasing your calorie intake is not necessarily the key. You must eat small amounts of certain recommended foods, and exercise regularly.

Q. *Are all carbohydrates fattening?*

A. Most complex-sugar carbohydrates are not fattening when eaten in moderate amounts.

Q. *Can you take too many vitamins?*

A. Indeed you can. Excessive doses of some vitamins can be dangerous. If you eat fresh, unprocessed, "non-junk" foods, you will get your normal supply of vitamins.

Q. *Are all "health" foods good for you?*

A. Some health foods substitute one harmful food for another; for instance, honey is often used instead of sugar, and "sea salt" may replace "ordinary" salt. Actually, "sea salt" and regular table salt are the same in sodium content. Some health foods, though possibly overpriced, are excellent. Read the labels carefully.

Q. *Do female hormones contribute to a woman's weight problems?*

A. Yes, usually they do. The female hormones estrogen and progesterone produce and store fat.

Q. *Do fat children tend to become fat adults?*

A. Unfortunately, yes. Once the pattern of overeating and underexercising is formed, it is difficult to change.

Q. *Is obesity usually a hormonal problem?*

A. No. Hormonal problems that cause obesity occur less than 5 percent of the time.

Q. *Why is it a good idea to eat slowly?*

A. The faster you eat, the more you will eat, and the faster your insulin will act on sugar and use it to manufacture fat.

Q. *Is it better to eat only one large meal instead of three small ones?*

A. No. Two or three small meals will cause less insulin to be secreted than one large meal. The extra insulin secreted during a large meal helps to manufacture fat from sugar.

Q. *Do men use up more calories than women do?*

A. Yes. A man's extra muscle tissue burns off twice as many calories as the more fatty body make-up of a woman.

Q. *Why do most women gain weight just before their monthly period starts?*

A. Weight gain just before the menstrual period begins occurs because the body retains extra fluid at that time. Fluid retention can be counteracted somewhat by avoiding salt, but a temporary weight gain is probably inevitable.

Q. *Do Americans get enough protein?*

A. It has been estimated that most Americans get about 10 percent *more* protein than their bodies need. People in the United States make up about 7 percent of the world's population, but consume about 30 percent of the world's meat supply.

Q. *Are nuts fattening?*

A. All nuts contain some fat. Almonds and filberts are relatively low in fat, and Brazil nuts, cashews and macadamia nuts are very high in fat.

Q. *Isn't a vegetarian diet basically incomplete and therefore unhealthy?*

A. As long as a vegetarian's diet is well-balanced, there is no reason to think of it as incomplete or unhealthy.

Q. *Why is it necessary to include exercise in a permanent diet program?*

A. Without some physical activity you will probably have trouble using up all the calories you eat.

Q. *Doesn't exercise stimulate the appetite?*

A. No. Exercise *decreases* your appetite because blood moves away from your stomach to the more active muscles, where the oxygen in the blood is needed.

Q. *What is the safest exercise?*

A. Walking.

Q. *Are salt tablets necessary after exercise, especially on hot, humid days?*

A. No. Your food contains enough natural salt to replenish the salt you lose when you perspire.

Q. *Are some people born with lower metabolisms than other people?*

A. It is true that people use up their calories at different rates.

Q. *Is it possible to change your metabolism?*

A. Most overweight people originally had normal metabolisms, which were disrupted by overeating. It may be difficult, but your metabolism can be changed again.

Q. *Does everyone digest food differently?*

A. The process of digestion is basically the same for everyone.

Q. *Why do people usually lose more weight during the first week of dieting than any other time?*

A. Weight loss during the first week of a diet usually consists of a great amount of fluid.

Q. *Why is vegetable oil recommended?*

A. Vegetable oils (such as corn oil and safflower oil) are low in saturated fats, which probably contribute to heart disease. In addition, many oils and shortenings are "hydrogenated" to slow the spoiling process. Liquid vegetable oils are not hydrogenated. This is another point in favor of vegetable oils, since hydrogenation destroys essential fatty acids and makes it difficult for the body to metabolize some oils. All oils will spoil faster in tins or plastic containers than in glass bottles.

Q. *Should a person on a diet eat low-fat yogurt or regular yogurt?*

A. Choose the yogurt that tastes best to you, as long as it is nonflavored. Regular yogurt contains about 3 percent fat, and so-called "low-fat" yogurt has almost 2 percent fat. The difference in fat content is so slight you don't need to be rigid about which type you eat.

Q. *Why shouldn't dieters eat poultry skin?*

A. Poultry skin contains high amounts of fat and salt.

Q. *Why is only water-packed tuna fish recommended?*

A. Some tuna fish is packed in oil, which is high in calories.

Q. *Is cholesterol harmful or not?*

A. Very high levels of cholesterol are definitely harmful. However, results of the Framingham study have shown that high levels of cholesterol may be offset by the presence of high-density lipoproteins (HDL) in the blood. When the level of HDL is high, the risk of elevated cholesterol is much less than when high levels of low-density lipoproteins (LDL) are present. Elevated cholesterol levels are not *necessarily* linked to a high-cholesterol diet, since the body manufactures its own cholesterol, especially in tense, high-strung people. Also, we know that the levels of HDL are high in individuals who engage in regular physical activity; marathon and long-distance runners have very high levels of HDL.

Chapter 10

The Rechtschaffen Recipes*

You are about to embark on a new way of life. You are going to deprive yourself of two important seasonings that you have been enjoying all your life—salt and sugar—and of the two of these, salt is the one likely to be missed more.

At first you may feel that your food is intolerably bland and uninteresting without salt, but it won't be long before you will become aware of nuances and subtleties of flavors that you never knew existed. They were always there, but were disguised by the killing flavor of salt.

As your palate gradually becomes "desalted," dishes will become more exciting and appetizing than ever before, and you will find heavily salted foods almost unpalatable.

*Note that most of the recipes produce enough food for four people. If you plan to make a single portion for yourself, reduce the quantities appropriately.

Use the Best
Ingredients and Cook
Them Carefully

The flavor has to be in the ingredients you put into a dish if you are going to taste it. It is therefore important to shop carefully and to buy only strictly fresh vegetables, chicken, fish and salad greens.

How the food is cooked is also important. Be careful not to overcook or undercook. Vegetables are best lightly steamed until barely fork-tender, and pastas should be cooked only until *al dente,* or "firm to the tooth."

As the weeks fly by, you will gradually see wonderful changes in your body. You will discover new vigor, a greater zest for living. Your sense of taste will become markedly sharper, and chances are you will want to reach out for more diversified and varied menus; you will want to try dishes that you never cooked or ate before. You will be more interested in quality and different taste sensations than in quantity. You will find yourself planning, shopping and preparing food more carefully, because cooking for a true food-lover becomes an experience to look forward to at the end of a busy day—a challenging, relaxing, rewarding hobby.

Flavor
hcighteners

At the start of your low-salt, low-simple-sugar, low-fat diet you may welcome a few tricks to heighten the flavor of your meals and make them more palatable.

Pepper

Investigate and experiment with various types and grinds of peppers. There are black peppercorns, finely ground, medium ground or coarsely cracked. Use them lavishly in salads and on chicken. Freshly ground white peppercorns have a very different, elusive flavor on fresh vegetables and fish and in veal dishes, while the many varieties of red pepper, cayenne, hot paprika, chili petines, hot pepper flakes, and fresh chili peppers in season, seeded and chopped, add sparkle to almost any bland dish. Then there are those intriguing green peppercorns, packed in water or vinegar, that make an excellent addition to grilled meats or chicken.

Other condiments

Homemade mustard—just dry mustard mixed to a paste with water or white wine—gives most dishes a sizable boost. So, too, do freshly grated horseradish and ginger root, both available frequently in the fresh food section of local markets. If they're not, you can buy powdered horseradish and reconstitute it in water or vinegar and use dried ginger root, whole or ground. (Prepared mustard may be used as long as it contains no additives.)

Herbs and spices

Use a variety of dried herbs in winter, fresh in summer if available, more frequently and in great, even daring, amounts.

Nutmeg enhances chicken dishes and braised spinach. A dash of cinnamon is a rather startling enhancer for veal and chicken. Try it also on your breakfast bran or shredded wheat.

Dill weed, tarragon and oregano are all lovely herbs to use generously, while thyme, rosemary and sage should be added with more caution.

Citrus fruits

Lemon or lime juice is good on most fish dishes, and grated zest of lemon, orange and lime are excellent additions to veal or chicken. Most vegetables, especially Brussels sprouts, broccoli, cauliflower and cabbage are enhanced by a generous squeeze of lime or lemon juice, and orange or grapefruit sections are occasionally used to garnish fish dishes or curries.

Buttermilk and yogurt

No-salt-added buttermilk and plain yogurt are almost essential ingredients in the Rechtschaffen Diet. Use buttermilk in soups and salad dressing; yogurt takes the place of butter or sour cream on such vegetables as baked potato, acorn or butternut squash, and is rather an exotic addition to a serving of hot spaghetti or rice.

Assertive vegetables

Pungent salad greens, such as arugula, watercress or Belgian endive, need little more than a simple dressing of vinegar or lemon juice and vegetable oil. Perk up the flavor of more delicate salad greens with chopped scallions or green pepper, sliced radishes, cucumber, zucchini or mushrooms. And don't forget the minced garlic!

Garlic

Use nothing but fresh garlic cloves—no dried garlic powder, and no garlic press, either. Smash a clove on your work surface with the side of a heavy knife, lift away the peel then chop through the clove every which way—presto—minced garlic.

Too high heat destroys the true flavor of garlic, making it bitter. Never put garlic under the broiler heat or sauté it in oil that's too hot. Generally it is best to add garlic to the liquid in a sauce, stew or soup just a few minutes before the dish is to be served.

Tomatoes

Salt-free tomatoes are available in cans when fresh tomatoes are out of season. Better yet, when they are in season, peel some red ripe tomatoes, chop and sauté a skilletful in a small amount of vegetable oil. Pack in freezer bags in appropriate amounts for your personal use and freeze.

Tomatoes, fresh or canned, are a great accompaniment to fish, chicken, pasta, rice, beans and on potatoes or bland vegetables, plain or mixed with yogurt.

On Mexican tables, a fresh tomato hot sauce will be found any time of the day or night. The following recipe is from

Diana Kennedy's *The Cuisines of Mexico,* which has become a classic in the world of cookbooks.

In her book, Diana writes that the sauce goes well with roasted or broiled meats or tacos. "It is marvelously crunchy and refreshing served just with tortillas. The Sinaloa version calls for some scallions and lime juice in place of the onions and water, and the Yucatecan version substitutes Seville orange juice for the water." Here is her recipe without the ½ teaspoon salt she uses—which you'll never miss!

SALSA MEXICANA CRUDA (FRESH MEXICAN SAUCE)

Makes about 1½ cups

    1 medium tomato (about 6 ounces)
    ½ medium onion
    6 sprigs fresh coriander
    3 chilies, preferably serranos
    ⅓ cup cold water

Chop all the ingredients finely—do not skin the tomato or seed the chilies. Mix together in a bowl and add the water.

Although this can be made up to three hours ahead, it is best made at almost the last minute, for it soon loses its crispness and the coriander its sharp flavor.

If you are unable to buy fresh coriander, I don't think Diana would mind very much if you used ¼ teaspoon ground coriander—but it would not be as flavorful.

The Recipes

Appetizers

BABA GHANNOUJ ((Eggplant Dip)

A delicious spread that makes an excellent lunch, especially because it may be kept in the refrigerator for several days. Serve with raw vegetables, whole-grain French bread, pita bread or low-salt matzoh crackers.

1 large eggplant
Juice of 1 lemon
1 tablespoon tahini or sesame paste
1 large clove garlic, minced
2 tablespoons chopped parsley
2 tablespoons olive oil

1. Cut stem and green hull from top of eggplant. Bake in 400° oven for about one hour, or until very soft. Scoop pulp out of skin and mash thoroughly or press through a sieve.
2. Slowly beat lemon juice into eggplant alternately with sesame paste. Stir in garlic.
3. Pile into serving bowl and garnish with chopped parsley. Sprinkle with olive oil.
   Yield: 4 servings
   Note: Some people like to sprinkle crushed red pepper on top.

PINEAPPLE WATERCRESS COCKTAIL

2 cups unsweetened pineapple juice
1 cup watercress leaves
2 tablespoons lemon juice
1 cup cracked ice

1. Put all ingredients into container of blender and blend on
    high speed for 20 seconds.
    Yield: 4 6-ounce cocktails

MARINATED GREEN BEANS AND
CHERRY TOMATOES

1 pound green beans, Frenched
1 dozen cherry tomatoes, halved
1 small onion, minced
1 tablespoon red wine vinegar
¼ teaspoon dry mustard
¼ teaspoon freshly ground pepper (preferably white)
3 tablespoons olive or vegetable oil
2 tablespoons minced parsley

1. Cook green beans in covered heavy saucepan with a small amount of water or steam until barely fork-tender.
2. Drain beans and empty into serving dish.
3. Add remaining ingredients, toss lightly, and marinate at room temperature until ready to serve. If made a day in advance, keep cold but remove from refrigerator at least 2 hours before serving.
   Yield: 4 servings

STUFFED MUSHROOMS

8 large mushroom caps
8 ounces low-salt, low-fat cottage cheese or pot cheese
2 tablespoons chopped chives
Freshly ground black pepper to taste
4 tablespoons yogurt
1 teaspoon lemon juice

1. Remove stems from mushrooms and reserve for soup stock. Rinse mushrooms and dry on absorbent paper.
2. Combine remaining ingredients and pile into mushroom caps. Chill until serving time.
   Yield: 4 servings

LENTILS WITH FRENCH DRESSING

¾ cup lentils
Pepper to taste
⅓ cup olive oil
2 tablespoons wine vinegar
2 tablespoons chopped scallions
¼ cup chopped parsley

1. Wash and pick over lentils. Simmer in 2 cups water for 30 to 40 minutes, or until tender.
2. Drain and combine with remaining ingredients. Serve at room temperature.
   Yield: 4 servings

CHICKPEAS RÉMOULADE

1½ cups cooked garbanzos, or chickpeas
4 tablespoons Blender Mayonnaise (page 176)
½ teaspoon dry mustard
¼ teaspoon coarsely cracked pepper
Lemon juice to taste
Shredded lettuce or romaine

1. Combine chickpeas, mayonnaise, spices and lemon juice.
2. Serve on a bed of shredded lettuce or romaine.
   Yield: 4 servings

BROILED MUSHROOMS

8 large fresh mushrooms
1 clove garlic, minced
2 teaspoons fresh chopped parsley or spinach leaves
2 teaspoons chopped chives or scallion tops
1 tablespoon chopped fresh dill or tarragon, or 1 teaspoon
   crumbled dry herb
1 tablespoon wine vinegar
¼ cup vegetable oil
Freshly ground black pepper to taste

1. Remove stalks from mushrooms and reserve for soup stock.
   Wash mushrooms if necessary and dry on absorbent paper.
2. Combine remaining ingredients. Fill mushroom caps with
   mixture and arrange in small baking dish.
3. Broil 5 inches from source of heat until mushrooms are
   hot.
   Yield: 4 servings

Soups

The basis of most good soups is a savory stock made of chicken, beef or veal with vegetables and herbs. Canned stocks and consommés are prohibited on this diet, not only because of their salt content but because their flavor is derived mainly from monosodium glutamate rather than from a complete protein food.

If you wish to make your own stock you may. Follow any recipe for stock, omitting the salt. Do not use any celery or foods on the "foods to avoid" list. Cool the broth or stock and chill it promptly. Then remove every speck of fat that will have congealed on the surface. Freeze in ice-cube trays. When frozen, empty the frozen cubes into plastic refrigerator bags to use when needed for soup or sauce.

Many excellent soups, however, are made with just plain water. These are known in France as *maigre* soups, or lean soups, and that's our goal, isn't it? One such example is the famous French onion soup served in Paris markets.

ONION SOUP

4 large sweet onions
3 tablespoons vegetable oil
2 cloves garlic, minced
4 cups water
Juice of ½ lemon
Freshly ground pepper to taste
Small loaf French bread

1. Peel and thinly slice onions.
2. In saucepan heat oil. Add onions and garlic and stew over medium heat for about 15 minutes, or until onions are wilted and transparent but not browned, stirring often to separate onion slices into rings.
3. Add water, lemon juice and pepper. Bring to a boil and simmer for 30 minutes. Correct seasoning.
4. Meanwhile slice French bread, place on baking sheet, and toast in a hot oven or under broiler heat until golden on both sides.
5. Ladle soup into plates and top each serving with a couple of slices of the toast.
   Yield: 4 servings

GARDEN SOUP

10 ripe tomatoes, quartered
1 medium onion, sliced
Handful of parsley sprigs
1 bay leaf
1 teaspoon peppercorns
4 cloves garlic
Dash allspice
½ lemon, sliced
½ cup each shredded raw carrots and green pepper
Unflavored yogurt

1. Into large saucepan put tomatoes, onion, parsley, bay leaf, peppercorns, garlic, allspice and lemon slices. Bring to a boil and simmer for 30 minutes. Discard lemon slices.
2. Press through fine sieve or strain to remove peppercorns and cloves, and blend to smooth purée in electric blender.
3. Into purée stir shredded vegetables.
4. Serve hot with a topping of yogurt on each serving.
   Yield: 4 servings

BARLEY SOUP

½ cup quick-cooking pearl barley
4 cups salt-free vegetable stock or water
2 large onions, chopped
2 tablespoons olive oil
½ cup chopped fresh mint
2 tablespoons chopped parsley
White pepper to taste
1 pint yogurt at room temperature

1. In saucepan combine barley and stock or water. Bring to a boil and simmer for 30 minutes, or until barley is tender.
2. While soup is cooking, sauté onions in oil until transparent. Add to soup along with mint, parsley and pepper, and simmer for 30 minutes longer.
3. Five minutes before serving, remove from heat, let stand 3 minutes, then stir in yogurt mixed with a little of hot broth.
    Yield: 4 servings

GAZPACHO

2 firm slim cucumbers
1 large sweet Bermuda onion
2 green peppers
8 red ripe tomatoes
2 large cloves garlic
6 tablespoons wine vinegar
¼ cup olive oil
½ teaspoon coarsely cracked pepper
1½ cups ice water
2 slices whole-wheat bread
2 tablespoons vegetable oil

1. Peel, seed and finely dice 1 cucumber. Peel and finely chop half onion. Seed and sliver 1 green pepper. Peel, quarter, squeeze out seeds and chop 6 tomatoes. Mince garlic.
2. Combine these prepared vegetables in bowl or pitcher and stir in vinegar, olive oil, pepper and water. Chill for several hours.
3. Prepare garnish: Peel, seed and dice remaining cucumber. Chop remaining onion. Seed and chop remaining green pepper. Peel, seed and chop remaining tomatoes. Put each vegetable in separate bowl and refrigerate.
4. Cut bread into cubes and brown lightly in vegetable oil. Drain on absorbent paper.
5. To serve, stir soup well and ladle into soup plates. Put an

ice cube in the center of each plate and pass chopped
vegetables and croutons separately.
Yield: 6 servings

●◄●◄●

CUCUMBER SOUP

4 firm slim cucumbers
2 pints unflavored yogurt
1 cup low-fat milk
2 tablespoons lemon juice
2 cloves garlic, minced
2 tablespoons chopped chives or fresh dill
Peppercorns

1.   Peel and seed cucumbers. Shred 3 cucumbers and combine
     with yogurt and milk. Stir in lemon juice, garlic and chives
     or dill.
2.   When ready to serve, shred remaining cucumber. Serve
     with an ice cube in the center of each serving, garnish with
     shredded cucumber, and pass the pepper grinder.
     Yield: 4 servings

Poultry

SOUTHERN FRIED CHICKEN
(¼ egg per serving)

The coating on this chicken stays so crisp that it is as good cold the next day as it is the day it is fried. You will not miss the salt. Use the highest quality, freshest chicken you can buy.

3- to 3½-pound frying chicken, cut into serving portions
1 egg
2 tablespoons cold water
½ teaspoon cracked peppercorns
½ cup unbleached flour
Vegetable oil for shallow frying

1. Wash and dry chicken parts. Remove skin and excess fat.
2. Beat egg with water and pepper in mixing bowl. Add chicken and let stand at room temperature for a few minutes, turning occasionally to coat pieces on all sides with egg mixture.
3. Measure flour into heavy paper bag. Add chicken pieces, and shake bag, holding it closed at the top, to coat chicken lightly with flour.
4. Heat enough oil in large chicken fryer or skillet to cover bottom by ¼ inch. (You will not use all this oil and can strain it into a container to use again.) Heat oil to very hot, but not smoking. Place pieces of chicken in it and fry for 5 minutes, or until nicely brown. Turn and brown other

side 5 minutes longer. Turn chicken again, reduce heat to medium, cover pan tightly and cook for 8 to 10 minutes, or until chicken is cooked to taste.

5. Drain chicken on paper towels, then transfer to serving platter and keep warm in a 200° oven until ready to serve.
Yield: 4 servings

BROILED ROCK CORNISH GAME HENS

2 Rock Cornish game hens, halved (use the fresh bird if possible)
2 tablespoons vegetable or olive oil
½ teaspoon coarsely cracked black pepper
Grated rind and juice of 1 lemon
1 large clove garlic, minced
1 teaspoon dry tarragon, crumbled

1. Put birds in a glass or plastic bowl and add remaining ingredients. Cover and marinate in refrigerator for 4 hours, or overnight, turning birds at least once.

2. When ready to cook, place birds skinside down on broiler rack and broil at least 6 inches from moderate heat for 15 minutes, watching that they do not burn. Turn, baste with marinade in bowl and broil for 15 minutes longer.
Yield: 4 servings

CHILI CON POLLO

3½- to 4-pound roasting chicken, quartered
1½ cups salt-free broth or water
2 1-pound cans salt-free whole tomatoes
4 tablespoons chili powder
1 teaspoon ground cumin
1 teaspoon oregano
2 cloves garlic, chopped
2 cups chopped onions
4 tablespoons unbleached flour
4 tablespoons water
Juice of ½ lemon

1. Wash and dry chicken and discard skin. Put into heavy kettle with broth or water, tomatoes, chili powder, cumin and oregano. Bring liquid to a boil.
2. Add garlic and onions, partially cover, and simmer over low heat for 1½ hours, or until chicken is very tender.
3. Remove chicken from broth with slotted spoon, discard bones and cut meat into large pieces.
4. In small bowl combine flour, 4 tablespoons water and juice of ½ lemon. Bring liquid in kettle to a rolling boil. Gradually stir flour mixture into liquid and cook, stirring, until sauce is thickened.
5. Return chicken to kettle, reduce heat and cook for 10 minutes longer. Serve with cooked couscous or rice.
   Yield: 4 servings

TURKEY PICCATA

Half a 2-pound turkey breast
2 to 4 tablespoons vegetable oil
1 shallot or scallion, finely chopped
Freshly ground pepper to taste
Juice of 2 lemons
Green peppercorns (water- or vinegar-packed)

1. Skin and bone turkey breast. Place in freezer for 1 hour, or until firm, but not frozen. Slice thin.
2. In large skillet heat oil and in it sauté turkey slices for about 3 minutes on each side, or until lightly brown. When brown, transfer to heated platter, sprinkle with pepper and keep warm. Continue browning remaining turkey slices, adding more oil if needed.
3. When all turkey is brown, turn heat to low and add shallot or scallion to juices remaining in skillet. Sauté, stirring, for 1 minute. Stir in lemon juice and cook, scraping pan to incorporate juices and brown bits of glaze into sauce. Pour over turkey slices and garnish with green peppercorns.
Yield: 4 servings

CHICKEN À L'ORANGE

2 whole chicken breasts, boned, halved and skinned
¼ cup unbleached flour
½ teaspoon paprika
1 teaspoon grated orange peel
2 tablespoons vegetable oil
1 clove garlic, minced
¼ cup white wine
½ cup orange juice
Pinch of thyme
1 orange, thinly sliced

1. Pound chicken breasts between pieces of waxed paper until thin.
2. In paper bag combine flour, paprika and orange peel. Add chicken, close bag at top, and shake to coat chicken with flour mixture.
3. In skillet heat oil and in it brown chicken breasts lightly on both sides. Transfer to shallow baking dish.
4. To skillet add garlic and cook, stirring, for 1 minute. Add wine, orange juice and thyme. Heat to boiling and pour over chicken.
5. Bake in preheated 350° oven for 15 minutes. Top with orange slices and continue to bake for 15 minutes longer.
6. Serve with rice.
   Yield: 4 servings

CHICKEN SAUTÉ HUNTER STYLE

2½- to 3-pound chicken, cut into serving pieces
Freshly ground black pepper
3 tablespoons vegetable oil
¼ pound mushrooms, wiped, trimmed and sliced
1 tablespoon chopped shallots or scallions
1 teaspoon flour
¼ cup dry white wine or dry vermouth
1 cup skinned, seeded, chopped tomato
1 tablespoon chopped parsley

1. Wash chicken pieces and dry on absorbent paper. Discard skin and sprinkle meat lightly with pepper.
2. In skillet heat 2 tablespoons of cooking oil. Arrange chicken in hot oil and cook over moderate heat for about 10 minutes, or until nicely brown. Turn and cook for 10 minutes, or until brown, on other side.
3. Add mushrooms and shallots, cover and cook for 10 minutes longer, or until chicken and mushrooms are tender.
4. Remove chicken from skillet to warm platter, cover with foil and keep warm. Add remaining tablespoon oil to skillet and sprinkle with flour. Cook, stirring, for 1 minute.
5. Add wine or vermouth, and cook until wine is reduced to half. Stir in tomato, and cook for 5 minutes. Correct seasoning with pepper.
6. Pour sauce over chicken and sprinkle with chopped parsley.
Yield: 4 servings

Meat

VEAL CHOPS IN WHITE WINE SAUCE

2 veal chops, about 8 ounces each
3 tablespoons vegetable oil
6 large fresh mushrooms, trimmed and sliced
Coarsely cracked pepper
½ cup dry white wine
2 tablespoons dry sherry or Madeira
1 teaspoon cornstarch mixed with 1 tablespoon water

1. Sauté veal chops in hot oil for about 3 minutes on each side, or until lightly browned.
2. Sprinkle mushrooms around chops and cook for 5 minutes, shaking pan frequently to toss mushrooms in oil.
3. Add pepper, white wine, sherry or Madeira. Cover and braise over low heat for 5 to 10 minutes longer.
4. Remove chops to serving platter and keep warm.
5. Stir cornstarch mixture into liquid in pan and cook, stirring, for 1 minute, or until sauce is slightly thickened. Pour sauce and mushrooms over chops and garnish with parsley or watercress.

Yield: 2 servings

VEAL POLONAISE

1½ pounds veal scallops or 4 thin slices cut from the leg
Pepper
Flour
2 fresh ripe tomatoes or a 1-pound can unsalted whole
   tomatoes
3 tablespoons vegetable oil
1 small onion, minced
⅓ cup dry white wine
1 tablespoon chopped parsley
½ cup unflavored yogurt
Parsley clusters for garnish

1. Pound slices of veal between two pieces of waxed paper
   with side of heavy cleaver or meat pounder until very thin.
   Sprinkle lightly with pepper and coat with flour.
2. Peel, seed and chop fresh tomatoes, or drain, seed and chop
   if canned tomatoes.
3. In skillet heat oil and in it sauté scallops for 2 to 3 minutes
   on each side, or until lightly browned.
4. Arrange meat on warm serving platter.
5. Add minced onion to oil in pan and sauté until transparent.
   Add tomatoes and cook, stirring, for 2 to 3 minutes.
6. Stir in white wine and parsley and boil until liquid is
   reduced to half. Stir in yogurt and heat to serving temperature.
7. Pour sauce over meat and garnish with parsley clusters.
   Yield: 4 servings

VEAL PAPRIKA

1½ pounds veal scallops or 4 thin slices cut from the leg
Freshly ground pepper
Flour
3 tablespoons olive oil
2 tablespoons vegetable oil
2 shallots or scallions, chopped
1 tablespoon paprika
¼ cup dry white wine
¼ cup salt-free broth or water
8 ounces unflavored yogurt

1. Pound slices of veal between two pieces of waxed paper with side of heavy cleaver or meat pounder until very thin. Sprinkle with pepper and coat lightly with flour.
2. In skillet heat olive oil and in it sauté scallops for 2 to 3 minutes on each side, or until lightly brown. Transfer meat to warm serving platter.
3. Add vegetable oil to juices in skillet and stir in shallots or scallions and paprika and sauté, stirring, for 30 seconds. Add wine and broth or water, and cook until liquid is reduced to half the quantity.
4. Gradually stir in yogurt and heat to serving temperature. Pour over meat.
   Yield: 4 servings

VEAL WITH TARRAGON

1½ pounds veal scallops or 4 thin slices cut from the leg
Pepper
Flour
4 tablespoons vegetable oil
8 mushrooms (½ pound), washed and sliced
2 shallots or ½ small onion, minced
½ cup dry white wine
1 teaspoon crumbled dry tarragon or 1 tablespoon chopped
    fresh
1 tablespoon minced parsley

1. Pound slices of veal between two pieces of waxed paper
    with side of heavy cleaver or meat pounder until very thin.
    Sprinkle them lightly with pepper and coat with flour.
2. In skillet heat 3 tablespoons oil and in it sauté veal over
    moderate heat for about 2 minutes on each side, or until
    lightly browned.
3. Transfer veal to warm platter. To oil remaining in pan add
    mushrooms and cook over low heat for 3 minutes, stirring
    frequently. Sprinkle mushrooms with shallots or onion and
    cook for 1 minute longer.
4. Add white wine and cook over high heat until liquid is
    reduced to half.
5. Add remaining tablespoon oil and swirl pan above the heat
    until sauce begins to simmer. Add tarragon and parsley and
    pour sauce over meat.
    Yield: 4 servings

Fish

SIZZLING FISH PLATTER WITH VEGETABLES

1½- to 2-pound whole fish (snapper, pompano
  or sea bass), ready to cook
1 lemon, thinly sliced
1 large onion, peeled and thinly sliced
2 ripe tomatoes, halved
1 green pepper, seeded and cut into strips
1 clove garlic, minced
3 tablespoons vegetable oil
½ teaspoon coarsely cracked pepper
Parsley and lemon wedges for garnish

1. Preheat oven to 400°. Oil large stainless steel or pewter platter.
2. Wash and dry fish. Make deep diagonal incisions on one side of fish, about 1 inch apart, and arrange lemon slices in the incisions. Squeeze any remaining lemon juice over fish.
3. Arrange onion, tomatoes and green pepper around fish. Sprinkle tomato halves with garlic and brush fish and vegetables with oil, dribbling it on tomatoes. Sprinkle with pepper.
4. Bake in preheated oven for 10 minutes. Reduce temperature to 350° and bake for 20 minutes longer, or until fish flakes easily.
5. Garnish platter with parsley clusters and lemon wedges.
  Yield: 2 servings

FILLETS OF SOLE OR FLOUNDER
WITH ALMONDS

4 fillets of sole or flounder (about 1½ pounds)
¼ cup unbleached flour
4 tablespoons vegetable oil
Freshly ground pepper to taste
½ cup blanched slivered almonds (unsalted)
Juice of ½ lemon
Watercress or parsley and lemon wedges for garnish

1. Carefully remove the fine line of bones that runs down the center of each fillet. Keep fish cold until ready to cook.
2. Spread flour on a piece of waxed paper. Coat fillets with flour and shake off all excess.
3. In skillet heat half the oil, and in it sauté fillets over moderate heat for 2 to 3 minutes on each side, or until lightly browned.
4. Remove fillets from pan to warm serving dish. Sprinkle lightly with pepper.
5. To skillet add remaining oil. As soon as it is hot, add almonds. Shake skillet back and forth until almonds are lightly toasted. Add juice of ½ lemon, and pour almonds and lemon oil over fish.
6. Garnish with watercress or parsley and lemon wedge. *Yield:* 4 servings

SKEWERED SWORDFISH

Use about ⅓ pound boneless fish steaks per person to be served. Cut steaks into cubes and marinate in vegetable oil seasoned with a little vinegar and pepper. Arrange cubes on skewers, alternating with slice of onion, wedge of tomato and bay leaf. Grill over burning coals, or under broiler heat, turning frequently, for about 5 minutes on each side. Slide fish from skewer onto serving plate and sprinkle with lemon juice.

GREY SOLE IN WHITE WINE

4 fillets of grey or lemon sole
6 shallots, chopped (2 to 3 tablespoons)
2 to 3 tablespoons chopped parsley
1 lemon
¼ cup dry white wine

1. Preheat oven to 375°.
2. Wash fillets and pat dry with absorbent paper.
3. Place fish in an ovenproof au gratin dish. Sprinkle with shallots and parsley. Squeeze juice of lemon over it.
5. Bake until sizzling hot, about 18 to 20 minutes, then pour enough white wine over it to moisten fish, about ¼ cup, and place under broiler for 3 to 5 minutes.

Yield: 4 servings

POACHED FILLET OF SOLE
WITH TOMATO SAUCE

4 fillets of sole or flounder
1 tablespoon vegetable oil
¾ cup dry white wine
2 tablespoons chopped onion
1 clove garlic, minced
2 tablespoons chopped parsley
2 large ripe tomatoes, peeled, seeded and chopped
1 tablespoon flour
2 tablespoons water
Pepper to taste
Parsley sprigs

1. Remove the fine line of bones that runs down the center of each fillet. Cut fillets in half lengthwise. Roll each half like a tiny jelly roll, and secure with a wooden pick.
2. Heat oil in skillet. Arrange fillets in pan, curled side up. Add wine, onion, garlic and parsley. Sprinkle with tomatoes.
3. Bring liquid to a simmer, cover skillet and let fish poach for 5 minutes. Turn and poach 5 minutes longer.
4. Transfer fillets with slotted spoon to warm serving platter and discard wooden picks.
5. Bring liquid remaining in skillet to a boil. Combine flour and water and stir into liquid. Season sauce with pepper and cook, stirring, for 2 minutes.

6. Pour sauce over the fillets and tuck a sprig of parsley into the center of each.

   Yield: 4 servings

FISH WITH ALMONDS AND BANANAS

4 fillets of sole or flounder or any white-fleshed fish
Flour
Pepper
3 tablespoons vegetable oil
2 bananas, halved lengthwise
½ cup unsalted blanched, slivered almonds
Juice of ½ lemon
2 tablespoons minced parsley

1. Coat fillets lightly with flour and sprinkle with pepper.
2. In skillet heat 2 tablespoons oil, and in it sauté fillets 3 to 4 minutes on each side, or until lightly brown and flesh flakes easily. Remove fillets to warm serving platter.
3. To skillet in which fish was fried, add remaining tablespoon oil, and in it sauté bananas for 2 to 3 minutes, or until delicately brown. Arrange half a banana on each fish fillet.
4. Add almonds to remaining oil in pan and sauté, stirring, until almonds are golden.
5. Stir in lemon juice and parsley and pour over fish.

   Yield: 4 servings

Pasta

FETTUCCINI WITH MUSHROOM SAUCE
(½ egg per serving)

½ cup vegetable oil
3 cloves garlic, chopped
1 pound fresh mushrooms, washed, trimmed and sliced
1 pound fettuccini, cooked and drained
½ teaspoon coarsely cracked black pepper or to taste
2 tablespoons chopped parsley

1. In saucepan or skillet combine oil, half the garlic and all the mushrooms. Cook over moderately high heat for 15 minutes, stirring occasionally.
2. Cook fettuccini *al dente* according to package instructions.
3. Pour over cooked hot fettuccini, sprinkle with pepper, remaining garlic and parsley and toss to mix.
Yield: 4 servings

SPAGHETTI WITH MARINARA SAUCE

2 tablespoons olive oil
1 large clove garlic, finely chopped
1 large (2 pound, 3 ounce) tin of Italian plum tomatoes
¼ can tomato paste
½ tablespoon basil
½ tablespoon oregano
1 pound spaghetti, preferably whole-grain, cooked and drained
1 tablespoon chopped parsley
Freshly ground black pepper

1. Heat oil in a heavy pot. Add peeled, chopped garlic and sauté for 5 minutes.
2. Press tomatoes a few at a time through sieve into garlic and oil mixture. Stir frequently. When all tomatoes have been pressed through sieve, add remaining ingredients—except spaghetti, parsley and pepper—and stir well.
3. Lower heat and simmer sauce for 45 minutes to 1 hour, stirring occasionally. Do not let sauce boil.
4. Cook spaghetti *al dente* according to package instructions.
5. Pour sauce over freshly cooked hot spaghetti, sprinkle with parsley and pepper.
Yield: 6 servings

SPAGHETTI WITH GARLIC AND OIL

This is a robust dish for garlic lovers. It's easy, yet tricky. The tricks are to slice the garlic paper-thin, and to cook it very slowly until just lightly toasted in the hot oil. If the garlic is permitted to overbrown, it becomes bitter.

¾ cup vegetable oil
10 to 12 large cloves garlic, peeled and sliced paper-thin
1 pound thin spaghetti, preferably whole-grain
Freshly ground black pepper

1. Heat oil in small skillet. Add garlic and place over moderate heat. Stand by. As soon as oil begins to bubble around edge of garlic slices, turn heat to low and cook, stirring occasionally, until garlic becomes crisp and pale gold. Remove from heat.
2. Meanwhile cook pasta in boiling water until *al dente.* Just before pasta is done, return garlic and oil to very low heat.
3. Drain pasta into a colander, and while still dripping wet, empty immediately into hot mixing bowl. Pour garlic and oil over pasta, and toss with wooden spoons, adding lots of freshly ground black pepper.
Yield: 4 servings

LINGUINE OR SPAGHETTI WITH BROCCOLI

1 bunch broccoli, about 1¼ pounds
6 tablespoons olive oil
2 teaspoons garlic, finely chopped
½ teaspoon crushed red pepper
½ cup chicken broth
Freshly ground black pepper
1 pound linguine or spaghetti, preferably whole-grain

1. Cut broccoli florettes off stems. Peel stems and cut into bite-size pieces. There should be about 6 cups of stem pieces and florettes.
2. Bring large pot of water to a boil and add broccoli. Cook about 1 to 3 minutes and drain. Do not overcook; broccoli must remain crisp. Run cold water over broccoli to chill quickly.
3. Heat oil in a skillet and add garlic. Cook briefly, without browning. Add broccoli and toss to heat through. Add crushed red pepper, broth and ground black pepper to taste, and bring to a boil.
4. Cook linguine or spaghetti *al dente* according to package directions.
5. Drain pasta and toss with hot broccoli mixture. Serve *immediately* on warm plates.
   Yield: 8 servings

Grains and Cereals

LEMON RICE

1½ cups water
1 cup rice
1 lemon
2 tablespoons vegetable oil
¾ cup "no-salt-added" buttermilk
Chopped parsley

1. In saucepan combine water and rice and bring to a rapid boil. Cover with tight-fitting lid, reduce heat to lowest possible, and cook for 20 minutes.
2. While rice is cooking, remove thin yellow peel from lemon and sauté it in oil for 3 minutes. Discard rind, add buttermilk and heat gently.
4. When rice is cooked and dry, remove cover and toss with fork. Stir in lemon-buttermilk mixture. Empty into serving dish and keep warm until ready to serve.
5. Sprinkle with parsley before serving.
   Yield: 4 servings

RISOTTO

2 tablespoons olive oil
1 small onion, chopped
1 cup rice
½ cup dry white wine
1½ cups water
1 teaspoon saffron threads (optional)
Pepper to taste

1. In heavy saucepan heat olive oil and in it sauté onion for 3 minutes, or until onion is transparent.
2. Add rice and cook, stirring, for 2 minutes, or until rice is well coated with oil.
3. Add wine, water and saffron. Bring liquid to a rapid boil. Cover tightly, reduce heat to very low, and cook for 20 minutes.
4. Remove cover and fluff rice with fork. Partially cover and keep over low heat until ready to serve. Toss again before serving and sprinkle with pepper.
   Yield: 4 servings

BARLEY PILAF

3 or 4 cloves garlic, peeled and chopped
2 medium onions, chopped
½ pound fresh mushrooms, washed, trimmed and sliced
¼ cup chopped fresh dill or 1 tablespoon dry dill weed
2 tablespoons vegetable oil
1 cup quick-cooking pearl barley
2¾ cups water
Juice of 1 lemon
½ teaspoon freshly ground black pepper

1. In 3-quart saucepan sauté garlic, onions, mushrooms and dill in oil for 3 to 4 minutes, stirring frequently.
2. Add remaining ingredients.
3. Bring water to a boil, reduce heat, cover and simmer for 25 minutes.
   Yield: 4 servings

MUSHROOM POLENTA

(¼ egg per serving)

½ cup corn meal
½ cup cold water
1½ cups boiling water
½ pound fresh mushrooms, trimmed and sliced
2 tablespoons vegetable oil
1 egg
1 tablespoon water
Wheat germ or additional corn meal
1 tablespoon olive oil

1. In small bowl or cup mix ½ cup corn meal to a smooth paste with cold water. Stir gradually into boiling water and cook, stirring constantly, until mixture is thick. Cover saucepan and cook over low heat for 10 minutes, stirring occasionally.

2. While corn meal is cooking, sauté mushrooms in vegetable oil for 5 minutes, or until tender, stirring frequently. Fold mushrooms into corn-meal mixture and pack into small loaf pan or 3-cup bowl.

3. Cool, cover with transparent film, and refrigerate for several hours or overnight.

4. When ready to use, turn polenta from pan or bowl and cut into slices ½-inch thick.

5. Beat egg lightly with water. Coat slices of polenta evenly

with the flour, dip into egg mixture, then roll in wheat germ or dry corn meal.
6. Sauté slices in olive oil for about 2 minutes on each side or until golden.
Yield: 4 servings

—‹—›—

BAKED GRITS
(¹⁄₆ egg per serving)

1 quart water
1 cup hominy grits
1 egg
1 cup low-fat milk

1. In saucepan bring water to a rapid boil. Gradually stir in grits and cook over moderate heat, stirring occasionally, for 1 hour. Cool.
2. Preheat oven to 400°. Oil a 2-quart casserole.
3. Stir egg and milk into hominy mixture, turn into prepared casserole and bake for 30 minutes.
Yield: 6 servings

BAKED BUCKWHEAT (KASHA)

2 tablespoons vegetable or olive oil
1 cup buckwheat groats (kasha)
Sprinkling of coarsely ground pepper
Dash nutmeg or cinnamon

1. Preheat oven to 400°.
2. In heavy skillet heat oil and in it cook kasha over moderate heat, stirring, for about 10 minutes.
3. Empty into casserole, and add enough boiling water to cover kasha by an inch. Cover and bake in preheated oven for 30 minutes.
4. Remove cover and add a little more water if kasha seems dry. Replace cover, reduce oven temperature to 300°, and bake for 30 minutes longer. Sprinkle with pepper and nutmeg or cinnamon.
Yield: 4 servings

BULGUR PILAF

1 medium onion, chopped
2 cloves garlic, chopped
2 tablespoons vegetable or olive oil
1 cup cracked wheat
½ cup dry white wine
1 cup water

1. Sauté onion and garlic in oil until transparent. Add cracked wheat, wine and water. Bring to a boil, cover tightly and cook over very low heat for about 1 hour, or until wheat is dry and cooked.
2. Fluff with a fork, partially cover and keep over low heat for a few minutes before serving.
   Yield: 4 servings

Vegetables

RAW VEGETABLES WITH
COTTAGE CHEESE AND YOGURT

½ cucumber
2 radishes
4 scallions
1 pimento
½ cup low-salt, low-fat cottage cheese
½ cup low-salt, low-fat natural plain yogurt
Freshly ground black pepper

1. Peel cucumber and discard seeds. Trim radishes and scallions.
2. Dice all the vegetables into a decorative soup bowl.
3. Add cottage cheese and yogurt.
4. Sprinkle generously with freshly ground black pepper.
5. Stir gently so vegetables mix with cottage cheese and yogurt.

   Yield: 1 serving
   Variation: Fresh chopped tomato may be added.

STEWED MIXED VEGETABLES

2 large onions, sliced
3 large tomatoes, sliced
1 eggplant, peeled and sliced
Pepper to taste
¼ cup chopped fresh coriander or Italian parsley
⅓ cup water
2 tablespoons olive oil
2 large cloves garlic, minced

1. In heavy saucepan arrange alternate layers of onion, tomatoes and eggplant, sprinkling each layer with pepper and chopped greens.
2. Add remaining ingredients, cover tightly, and simmer for about 30 minutes, or until liquid is reduced to a rich gravy. *Yield:* 4 servings

BROILED EGGPLANT

1 medium eggplant, cut lengthwise into 6 sections
1 clove garlic
½ teaspoon oregano
½ cup vegetable oil
1 tablespoon wine vinegar

1. Peel eggplant sections.
2. Crush garlic with oregano, oil and vinegar and brush on eggplant.
3. Broil under low heat, turning occasionally and basting with the flavorful oil, until fork-tender, about 15 minutes.
   Yield: 6 servings

POTATOES PAPRIKA

2 tablespoons vegetable oil
1 small onion, finely chopped
1 teaspoon sweet paprika
2 large potatoes, peeled and sliced ¼-inch thick
2 tablespoons vinegar
1 bay leaf
½ teaspoon freshly ground black pepper

1. In skillet heat oil and in it sauté onion until golden.
2. Stir in paprika.
3. Add potatoes, vinegar, bay leaf, pepper and enough water to barely cover the potatoes.
4. Cover skillet and cook over low heat for 30 minutes, or until potatoes are tender.
5. Serve pan sauce with potatoes.
   Yield: 4 servings

SHREDDED ZUCCHINI

For each person to be served, use 1 small, slim, firm zucchini, 1 scallion and 1 tablespoon vegetable oil. Shred zucchini on medium grater and slice scallion, including tender green part. In small skillet or wok, heat 1 tablespoon vegetable oil. Add zucchini and scallion and cook over moderate heat, stirring constantly, for 2 to 3 minutes. The length of time will depend on how coarsely the zucchini was shredded. Sprinkle with pepper and chopped parsley or fresh dill or tarragon.

CURRIED GREEN PEPPERS

Use 1 large fresh green pepper for each serving. Wash, discard stem and seeds and cut into thin strips.

In skillet heat 1 tablespoon oil. Add 1 clove garlic, minced, and 1 teaspoon curry powder. Cook, stirring, over moderate heat for 2 minutes. Add green pepper, cover and cook for 20 minutes over low heat, or until green pepper is just fork-tender, stirring occasionally. Serve with pan juices spooned over.

BROILED TOMATOES WITH GARLIC

4 large ripe tomatoes
Pepper
¼ cup wheat germ
1 clove garlic, minced
2 tablespoons chopped parsley
2 tablespoons olive oil.

1. Preheat oven to 450°.
2. Do not peel tomatoes. Wash and cut in half crosswise. Arrange halves, cut side up, on baking sheet and sprinkle with pepper.
3. Combine wheat germ with garlic, parsley and olive oil. Sprinkle tomatoes with wheat-germ mixture. Bake in hot oven for 10 minutes, or until topping is lightly browned and tomato is heated through.
   Yield: 4 servings

LENTIL CURRY

½ pound lentils (1 cup)
1 onion, chopped
3 cloves garlic, peeled and chopped
2-inch stick cinnamon
½ teaspoon turmeric
1 tablespoon lemon juice
3 cups water
1 tablespoon oil
½ cup buttermilk
Freshly ground black pepper to taste

1. Wash lentils in cold water. Put into saucepan and add half the onion, two cloves of garlic, cinnamon, turmeric, lemon juice and water. Bring to a boil and cook until lentils are soft and most of water has been absorbed.
2. In small skillet heat oil and in it sauté remaining onion and garlic until lightly brown. Stir into lentils along with buttermilk. Season to taste with pepper.
    Yield: 4 servings

GARDEN PEAS À LA FRANÇAISE

1 tablespoon vegetable oil
1½ pounds young green peas, shelled
1 small head lettuce, washed and shredded
8 small white onions, peeled
Pinch of thyme
1 tablespoon chopped parsley
½ teaspoon freshly ground white pepper

1. Heat oil in saucepan. Add peas, lettuce, onions, thyme, parsley.
2. Cover pan tightly and simmer over low heat for 10 minutes, or until peas are tender, adding a spoonful of water if necessary to keep peas from sticking. Season with pepper.

Yield: 4 servings

Salads and Dressings

Salads should be eaten frequently on the Rechtschaffen Diet, and there is no better salad for everyday enjoyment than the traditional green salad tossed with homemade French Dressing, or Sauce Vinaigrette.

Buy only the freshest salad greens and combine several varieties. One of the best combinations is the pungent Italian watercress known as arugala or roquette—available at Italian markets—mixed with slivers of Belgian endive. Other excellent salad greens are domestic watercress, tender leaves of field salad, oak leaf lettuce, Bibb lettuce, romaine, escarole, curly endive (chickory) and head lettuce.

The greens should be washed, dried, wrapped in a terrycloth towel and stored in the refrigerator until ready to use.

To the green salad may be added such flavor heighteners as chopped green pepper, sliced radishes or young zucchini, diced cucumber, peeled, seeded ripe tomato, chopped scallions, sliced fresh mushrooms, and so on, and any desired salad herb, fresh or dried.

The salad greens may be mixed in the salad bowl in advance, providing they are kept cold. The salad dressing should be added to the greens just before serving, and greens and dressing should be tossed just until every leaf is lightly coated with oil.

Safflower is the preferred oil. Mix it with olive oil in the proportion of 1 part olive to 3 parts safflower oil.

FRENCH DRESSING,
OR SAUCE VINAIGRETTE

¼ teaspoon freshly ground pepper
½ teaspoon dry mustard
1 tablespoon vinegar or lemon juice
4 tablespoons salad oil (one part olive)
1 clove garlic (optional)

1. In small bowl mix pepper and mustard with vinegar or lemon juice.
2. Gradually whip in salad oil.
3. The garlic may be used in either of two ways. Before putting salad greens in bowl, the bottom and sides may be rubbed with garlic clove, cut in half. Or it may be minced and added to salad dressing.
4. Set dressing aside until ready to use. Whip again lightly before pouring over salad.
   Yield: ⅓ cup, or enough for a green salad for 4.

BUTTERMILK DRESSING

¼ cup vegetable oil
1 small clove garlic, peeled
2 tablespoons wine vinegar
2 tablespoons yogurt
¼ cup buttermilk
Lemon juice to taste
2 scallions, chopped

1. Into blender container put oil, garlic, vinegar and yogurt. Cover and blend on high speed for 5 seconds. Remove cover, and with motor on, pour in buttermilk.
2. Remove container from blender and add lemon juice to taste. Stir in scallions.
   Yield: ¾ cup

MAKE YOUR OWN YOGURT

1 quart low-fat milk
1 cup instant dry milk powder
½ cup commercial yogurt (unflavored)

1. Pour milk into a heavy saucepan and bring to a boil. Watch carefully not to let it boil over the pan. Reduce heat and simmer for 5 minutes, stirring occasionally.
2. Remove from heat, stir in milk powder, and cool to lukewarm (110°).
3. Stir in yogurt. Cover saucepan with tight-fitting lid and wrap in heavy towel. Set into oven (heat off) for 6 to 8 hours, or overnight. Or, easier yet, pour lukewarm mixture into a wide-mouthed thermos and seal tightly until the next day.
4. Spoon yogurt into pint jars and chill.
   Yield: 1 quart

YOGURT DRESSING

8 ounces unflavored yogurt
1 tablespoon vegetable oil
1 tablespoon lemon juice or tarragon vinegar
½ teaspoon dry mustard
1 tablespoon chopped chives
1 clove garlic, minced
Freshly ground black pepper.

Combine all ingredients and leave at room temperature until ready to spoon onto cold salad greens.
Yield: 4 servings

COTTAGE CHEESE DRESSING

½ cup fresh tomato juice
¼ cup low-fat cottage cheese
1 tablespoon lemon juice
½ teaspoon curry powder

Put all ingredients into container of an electric blender and blend on low speed until smooth.
Yield: 4 servings

BLENDER MAYONNAISE
(⅕ egg per quarter cup)

1 egg
½ teaspoon dry mustard
2 tablespoons vinegar
1 cup salad oil

1. Break egg into blender container. Add mustard and vinegar.
2. Add ¼ cup of oil. Cover and turn motor on low speed.
3. Immediately remove cover and pour in remaining ¾ cup oil in a steady stream.
   Yield: 1¼ cups

Homemade mayonnaise may be flavored to taste with garlic or herbs or curry (preferably paste rather than powder). Lemon juice may be used instead of vinegar. Red or white wine vinegar or cider vinegar may be used.

———•——

SAUCE VERTE

(for poached or sautéed fish)

2 tablespoons cut chives
1 teaspoon dry tarragon
¼ cup parsley clusters
1 teaspoon dill weed
1¼ cups Blender Mayonnaise (page 176)

Stir to combine in blender container, cover, and blend on high speed for 10 seconds.

Yield: 1½ cups

MIXED VEGETABLE SALAD

4 ripe tomatoes, peeled, seeded and chopped
1 green pepper, seeded and chopped
1 cucumber, peeled, seeded and diced
1 bunch radishes, sliced
1 bunch scallions, including tender green part, sliced
¼ cup chopped parsley
2 cups shredded romaine
1 clove garlic, minced
Freshly ground pepper to taste
2 tablespoons lemon juice
⅓ cup olive oil

1. Combine vegetables in salad bowl. Sprinkle with pepper.
2. Add lemon juice and olive oil and toss lightly.
   Yield: 4 servings

TABOOLEY (Parsley and Bulgur Salad)

1 cup cracked wheat (bulgur)
1 cup chopped sweet onion
1½ cups chopped parsley
½ cup finely chopped fresh mint leaves
½ cup vegetable oil
¼ cup lemon juice
Freshly ground pepper to taste
Head of romaine lettuce
Peeled, chopped ripe tomato

1. Soak bulgur in just enough water to cover for 1 hour. Drain and press out excess moisture.
2. In salad bowl combine bulgur, onion, parsley, mint, oil, lemon juice and pepper. Chill.
3. Serve on a bed of romaine leaves garlanded with chopped tomato.
   Yield: 4 servings

CABBAGE AND CUCUMBER SALAD

½ medium head cabbage, cored and shredded
1 slim, firm cucumber, sliced
2 tablespoons oil
3 cloves garlic, mashed with a little of the oil
3 tablespoons lemon juice
6 radishes, sliced

1. In salad bowl combine all ingredients except radishes. Chill for at least 2 hours, tossing occasionally.
2. Just before serving, toss in the radishes.
   Yield: 4 servings

CHINESE CABBAGE SALAD

1 head Chinese cabbage
1 bunch scallions, chopped
1 cup sliced crisp radishes
¼ cup chopped parsley
Juice of ½ lemon
⅓ cup salad oil
Freshly ground pepper to taste

1. Wash cabbage and discard discolored leaves. Shred into salad bowl.
2. Add scallions, radishes and parsley. Toss with lemon juice, salad oil and pepper.
3. Chill for 1 hour before serving.
   Yield: 4 servings

GINGERED CUCUMBER SALAD

2 large cucumbers, peeled and thinly sliced
2 tablespoons red wine vinegar
2 tablespoons shredded fresh ginger root
2 tablespoons vegetable oil
Head of romaine lettuce

Combine all ingredients except romaine and chill. Serve on a bed of shredded romaine.
Yield: 4 servings

ORANGE AND ONION SALAD

2 large oranges
½ large purple onion
Bibb lettuce
2 tablespoons vinegar
1 teaspoon grated orange peel
¼ cup orange juice
Juice of ½ lemon
½ teaspoon dry mustard
⅓ cup salad oil

1. Peel oranges, remove all white pith and cut each into 6 slices.
2. Peel onion and slice very thin.
3. Wash Bibb lettuce thoroughly, shake dry and refrigerate.
4. Combine remaining salad dressing ingredients.
5. Put orange and onion slices in a bowl, pour salad dressing over them, and marinate for at least 4 hours at room temperature.
6. When ready to serve, arrange leaves of lettuce on individual salad plates, and put orange and onion slices on top.
   Yield: 4 servings

SPINACH SALAD

10 ounces fresh spinach
1 small onion, minced
1 tablespoon olive oil
1 clove garlic, minced
1 cup yogurt
2 tablespoons chopped toasted walnuts

1. Wash spinach thoroughly. Drain well and chop coarsely.
2. Cook spinach with onion in covered saucepan without additional moisture for 10 minutes, tossing occasionally. Drain again.
3. Add oil and cook, stirring, for about 3 minutes longer.
4. Turn into serving bowl and mix lightly with garlic and yogurt. Sprinkle with walnuts and chill. Serve cold.
   Yield: 4 servings

ZUCCHINI AND WATERCRESS SALAD

1 slim zucchini, sliced
1 bunch watercress leaves
1 tablespoon chopped sweet onion
1 tomato, peeled, seeded and chopped
1 tablespoon chopped fresh sweet basil
1 tablespoon chopped parsley
3 tablespoons French Dressing (page 173)

Combine all ingredients in salad bowl. Toss and serve.
Yield: 2 servings

Desserts

MELON AND BERRIES

Fill the cavity of a slice of melon with strawberries or other berries in season. Sprinkle with a little white wine or dry sherry and freshly grated ginger root.

CREOLE STRAWBERRIES AND PINEAPPLE

Combine equal quantities of fresh pineapple cubes and fresh strawberries. Moisten with a little orange juice.

STRAWBERRIES CARDINAL

Blend 1 pint fresh strawberries with ¼ cup dry white wine. Strain through a sieve and pour over 2 pints fresh strawberries. Sprinkle with blanched shredded almonds.

FRUIT CUP

Combine equal parts diced apples, pears and bananas. Sprinkle with lemon juice and a dusting of cinnamon.

ORANGE MINT COCKTAIL

Separate 4 small oranges into sections. Discard the thin membranes. Moisten with a little lemon or pineapple juice and garnish with a sprig of mint.

PAPAYA CUP

Arrange balls of ripe papaya in a fruit cocktail glass. Moisten with lime juice, top with papaya seeds and garnish with a sprig of mint.

SHERRIED MIXED FRUIT

4 large oranges
1 pineapple
2 tablespoons finely chopped mint
1 tablespoon lemon juice
1 tablespoon pineapple juice
¼ cup dry sherry
Mint sprigs

1. Cut away all rind and bitter white pith from oranges. Separate into segments.
2. Peel, core pineapple and cut into cubes.
3. Combine equal quantities of orange sections and pineapple cubes, and toss with mint, lemon juice, pineapple and sherry.
4. Serve in fruit cocktail cups garnished with sprigs of mint.

RAW APPLESAUCE

Core and coarsely cut, but do not peel, 2 large or 4 small tart apples. Put ⅓ of apple pieces into blender container with ½ cup pineapple or orange juice and 1 thin slice lemon with rind. Cover and blend on high speed. Uncover and, with motor on, gradually add remaining apples. Serve with unflavored yogurt if desired.

Yield: 2 cups

Appendix

What Are the Essential Nutrients?

All food is made up of various combinations of three main kinds of nutrients: carbohydrates, fats and proteins—plus water and vitamins and minerals. Starch and carbohydrates are often confused. Starch *is* a carbohydrate, and is, in fact, the most common carbohydrate in your diet. Some high-starch foods are rice, bread, potatoes and pasta.

Carbohydrates

Glucose (commonly called blood sugar) results from the breakdown of carbohydrates. Glucose is the body's main energy source, and provides about two thirds of the body's daily calorie requirement.

There are two kinds of sugars, complex and simple. Simple sugars are digested in your mouth, and are rushed into your bloodstream almost immediately. In contrast, complex sugars

—carbohydrates—are digested and absorbed slowly. Complex sugars provide a steady flow of useful energy for your body.

When you eat complex sugars, such as pasta, vegetables or whole-grain bread, you reach a normal level of satisfaction quickly, and you stop eating. Such an end-signal does not occur so easily when you eat simple sugars. Remember how you can eat pounds of candy without feeling full? You could not possibly eat as much bread without being satisfied.

A typical chocolate bar contains about 90 percent sugar, and as many calories as 3 to 4 slices of bread. (Some popular breakfast cereals contain more sugar than a candy bar.) In addition, the calories in simple sugars are turned into fat *twice* as quickly as complex sugars. This means that the bread you eat will be less fattening than candy.

Simple sugars—such as those found in candy, ice cream, cake and soft drinks—increase the blood insulin level quickly in order to use up the sugar that is pouring into your blood. This rapid chemical reaction also produces free fatty acids, which raise the fat content in the blood and increase the likelihood of fatty deposits on the walls of arteries. These deposits can eventually contribute to stroke, heart attack, or kidney disease.

Dr. John Yudkin, British expert on metabolism, says in his book *Sweet and Dangerous, "There is no physiological require-ment for [simple] sugar;* all human nutritional needs can be met in full without having to take a single spoon of white or brown or raw sugar, on its own or in any food or drink.... *If only a small fraction of what is already known about the effects of [refined simple] sugar were to be revealed in relation to any other material used as a food additive, that material would promptly be banned."*

The words to be careful about are "refined" or "simple,"

not "carbohydrate." The carbohydrates found in such foods as pasta, potatoes, whole-grain cereals (including whole-grain breads), peas, soybeans, corn and rice are highly recommended components of your diet—just don't smother them with butter, salt and cream sauces, or have huge portions. Complex sugars, including starches, provide energy, allow your body to use fats efficiently, and spare your protein for tissue building and repairing instead of diverting it as a major energy source.

To repeat. There are two kinds of sugars: 1) Complex sugars (including vegetables and starches) are recommended *in moderation*; 2) simple sugars can kill you slowly, and should be avoided.

Besides starches and sugars, carbohydrates are also found in celluloses, the usually fibrous foods such as bran and vegetables that provide the necessary bulk in your diet.

Fats

Fats are essential to provide energy, supply a natural cushion for sensitive areas of the body, help build cells and tissues, and aid the absorption of fat-soluble vitamins A, D, E and K. But let's face it, fats are fattening.

When fat is oxidized or "burned" inside your body, it releases 9 calories for each gram burned. Carbohydrates and proteins yield only 4 calories per gram. In other words, fats give you more than twice the calories of most other foods.

An important point about fat in foods is that you can't always see it. For instance, meat or nuts don't have to be visibly fatty to contain many fat-generated calories. Shrimp is a relatively low-calorie food, but even though there is no visible fat there is actually a great deal of cholesterol in shrimp.

There are many kinds of fats, but the three we need to be concerned about here are saturated, mono-unsaturated and polyunsaturated. Saturated fats *raise* the level of blood cholesterol, mono-unsaturated fats have no effect on cholesterol levels, and polyunsaturated fats actually *lower* your cholesterol level.

Proteins

Protein is made up of twenty amino acids that have been called the building blocks of the body, because they can be combined in almost unlimited combinations to create new cells and tissues to renew your body.

When you eat a veal cutlet, for instance, your body does not absorb *veal* proteins. Instead, your body breaks it down into amino acids, which are then absorbed and rearranged to make *your* unique proteins. Each person has a special genetic code for reassembling amino acids into his or her own specific proteins. The process works in the same way that a builder can build different types of houses using the same building materials.

Without proteins, your body would waste away and die. No new cells would form, and no oxygen could be carried through the blood by the protein hemoglobin. Digested protein eventually becomes skin, hair, fingernails, enzymes, hormones, the general tissues of the body, and antibodies that fight infection.

The body can make about half of the twenty amino acids you need, but the other half must be obtained from the food you eat. The amino acids your body cannot manufacture on its own are called *essential* amino acids and are found in abundance in meat, fish, chicken, eggs and dairy products. Soybeans, chickpeas and peanuts provide almost as much protein as the foods from animal sources, and even bread, cereal, fruits and vegetables contain some protein. Most Americans get more than enough protein, but vegetarians should be careful that they are not deprived of sufficient amounts.

Some high-protein foods such as eggs, beef, shellfish and pork also contain large amounts of cholesterol, fat and calories. Equally useful protein foods, like chicken, veal and fish are low in cholesterol, fat and calories.

A word of caution about proteins: As important as protein is, your body cannot survive on *only* protein, no matter what any "diet expert" may say. Make sure that your overall diet is well-balanced with fats and carbohydrates as well as proteins.

Water

Most of us tend to forget how important water is and how easy it is to get the maximum benefits from it. Did you know that you can live for weeks without food but only for a few days without water? Digestion and absorption would be impossible without water because nutrients in your food must be dissolved in water before they can be absorbed into your bloodstream. Water also helps regulate body temperature, carries waste products out of your body via the kidneys, and maintains the general health of your cells and tissues.

About two thirds of your body is made up of water, and this delicate balance must be maintained by a daily intake of water. Adults take in about two and a half quarts of water every day, most of it through the foods and liquids they eat and drink. Under normal conditions, the same amount of water is given off each day, mainly through perspiration, evaporation from the lungs, and urine excretion.

Almost half of the water you need comes from the liquids you drink. The rest is found in such "dry" foods as meat (50 to 70 percent water), fruits and vegetables (usually more than 90 percent water) and even cereals and bread (about 35 percent water).

Drink 4 to 6 glasses of water every day. Water is a great diet food because it acts as an appetite suppressant. It is your best nutrition bargain.

Vitamins

You get the vitamins you need from food because your body cannot manufacture them. Ordinarily, vitamins are required in tiny amounts, but their importance is enormous. Vitamins play such an important role in supporting the work of a number of enzymes that vitamin deficiencies cause many different diseases.

As you know, there are many controversies about the benefits or harmful effects of large doses of vitamins, and each year a new claim for a wonder vitamin is made. Vitamin C has captured most of the headlines because of its possible role in preventing colds, and because its most active champion is two-time Nobel prize winner Linus Pauling. But Vitamin E seems to be gaining some of the limelight because of its supposed power to enhance sexual performance.

Most people do not need extra vitamin supplements if they are eating a well-balanced diet. Where a vitamin deficiency is evident, your physician will doubtlessly prescribe the correct vitamin to restore the proper nutritional balance. These days, when many people are involved in the quest for perfect health, some people may even be getting too *much* of a vitamin rather than too little. Excessive doses of some vitamins can be quite harmful. Ordinarily, we should be most concerned about getting too much Vitamin A and D, which can cause sluggishness and skin problems.

Both B and C vitamins, being water soluble, are easily destroyed by cooking and processing. Obviously, cooking, canning and other processing cannot be avoided altogether, but you should be aware of the problem and try to conserve the natural vitamins in your food whenever possible. It has been reported that smoking may decrease the amount of Vitamin C that is absorbed into the blood and that too much alcohol may interfere with the absorption of some of the B vitamins.

Most physicians are willing to stand by two simple statements of advice about vitamins: 1) It does no harm to take a daily multipurpose vitamin that contains B-complex and C but does not contain A and D (you probably get enough A and D in your diet and from sunshine, respectively, and too much of these vitamins can be harmful); and 2) Just because one vitamin is good it doesn't mean that 2 or 4 or 10 will be better.

Eat well and you won't have to get hung up on vitamins.

Minerals

At least fourteen minerals are essential for the maintenance of a healthy body, and their benefits range from the development of good bone structure to the activation of enzymes.

As with vitamins, you probably receive all the minerals you need in a normal diet, and there is no reason to rush out and stock up on the current crop of fashionable minerals. (I recommend a zinc supplement because diets that are low in beef and high in residue may be low in this substance.) Women who are pregnant may need additional calcium and iron in their diets, but such a recommendation should always come from the attending physician.

Index

About the Authors

JOSEPH S. RECHTSCHAFFEN, M.D., did graduate work in endocrinology and organic chemistry before receiving his medical degree in internal medicine. Until recently he was Chief of Gastroenterology at Beckman Downtown Hospital in New York and also served on the staffs of Beth Israel and Flower Fifth Avenue hospitals. He remains on the staffs of Beekman and Doctors hospitals in New York and has a private practice specializing in gastroenterology and nutrition. He lives in New York City with his wife. The Rechtschaffens have three sons, two of whom are physicians, and the third a pre-law student at Berkeley; their daughter is a resident physician at Cambridge Hospital.

ROBERT CAROLA is a writer with extensive editorial and writing experience, and is the author (with Professor Donald D. Ritchie) of the highly praised *Biology*. He lives in Westport, Connecticut, with his wife and children.

ANN SERANNE has written, collaborated on, or edited some twenty cookbooks, including *Good Food & How to Cook It* and *The Blender Cookbook* (with Eileen Gaden).